Essential Guide to Perimenopause for Women Over 35

Navigating Hormonal Changes, Symptoms Relief, Strategies for Healthy Body Balance, and Thriving Through Midlife

Kristin Hampton

Copyright © 2024 by Kristin Hampton

Disclaimer

The only objective of this book is to provide information; it is not meant to be used as a source of medical prescriptions or recommendations. It is important to note that the material included in this book is derived from the author's own experiences, research, and views. It is not intended to serve as a replacement for the advice, diagnosis, or treatment offered by a qualified medical professional.

This book's author and publisher do not make any claims or guarantees on the truth, applicability, suitability, or completeness of the information included within it. They expressly disclaim all guarantees, whether explicit or implied, as well as any claims about merchantability or suitability for any individual purpose. It is not possible to hold the author or publisher responsible for any loss or harm that may occur as a result of the utilisation of the information that is included in this book.

While every effort has been taken to guarantee the accuracy of the material contained in this book, the author and publisher accept no responsibility for mistakes or omissions, or any consequences arising from the use of the information within.

About the Author

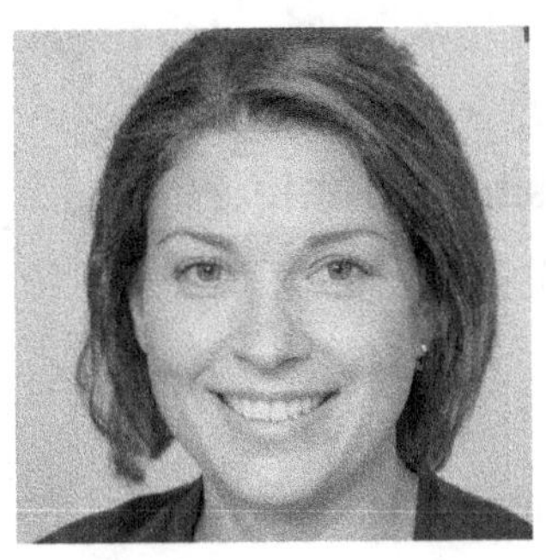 Kristin Hampton is a seasoned professional in the fields of holistic living, wellness, and beauty, with a wealth of experience and expertise to guide individuals on their journey to optimal health and radiant beauty. As a dedicated advocate, Kristin has devoted her career to empowering others to embrace holistic well-being and cultivate a lifestyle that nourishes both body and soul.

With a passion for research and a commitment to excellence, Kristin has become a trusted authority in the realm of wellness, offering practical insights and evidence-based strategies to help individuals thrive in today's fast-paced world. Through her captivating writing and engaging presentations, she shares her wealth of knowledge, drawing from her own experiences as well as the latest scientific research to provide actionable advice for sustainable health and wellness.

Beyond her professional achievements, Kristin is a devoted wife and mother, finding joy and fulfilment in the intricacies of family life. This steadfast dedication to her loved ones underscores her approach to wellness, emphasising the importance of balance, harmony, and self-care in every aspect of life.

Join Kristin on this transformative journey toward radiant living, and discover the true beauty that lies within.

Table of Contents

Introduction

Emily, a dynamic and accomplished lady in her early forties, had long taken delight in her deftness in switching between several responsibilities. On the other hand, she started to notice little changes when she reached perimenopause. A slight discomfort crept into her as she started to detect changes in her menstrual cycle, mood swings, and sleep problems. At first, she ignored the symptoms, thinking they were just minor setbacks. She continued to push through, blaming her hectic schedule and her will to keep moving forward.

Emily became more and more agitated and irritated as the months went by. Even the most mundane of duties became overwhelming, and she lost interest in things she used to like. A decline in Emily's mental health started impacting her relationships and productivity at work, even though she tried to hide her inner agony.

A friend of Emily's made a subtle observation about her pale skin and the lack of energy in her eyes one day at a social event. The impact of perimenopause on her mental and physical health became clear at that moment. She felt a renewed sense of urgency and set out to find information and people to help her cope with her problems.

Emily's path is not unusual. Many women encounter comparable issues during perimenopause, however, too often, they suffer in silence, ignorant of the tools available to assist them manage this transition.

This book is for any woman who finds herself at the crossroads of perimenopause, seeking direction, understanding, and empowerment. Whether you're just starting to notice the tiny indicators of hormonal changes or you're in the thick of navigating the rollercoaster of symptoms, remember that you can take control of your health and well-being.

Perimenopause, also referred to as the transition to menopause, signifies a key milestone in a woman's life, marking the steady loss of reproductive hormones and the approach of menopause.

But what precisely is perimenopause?
Perimenopause is a normal period in a woman's life, often commencing in her late 30s to early 40s, but the age of commencement may vary greatly among people. During this period, a woman's body experiences a series of hormonal swings as it prepares for the cessation of menstruation and the end of her reproductive years.

While menopause technically starts after a woman has gone 12 consecutive months without a menstrual cycle, perimenopause spans the years leading up to her last menstrual period. It's characterised by a variety of symptoms and changes, both physical and emotional, as the body adapts to altering hormone levels.

Symptoms of perimenopause may vary considerably from woman to woman, but some frequent experiences include irregular periods, hot flashes, night sweats, mood swings, trouble sleeping, vaginal dryness, and changes in libido. These symptoms may be disruptive and disturbing, influencing different elements of a woman's life – from her physical health and mental well-being to her relationships and general quality of life.

Perimenopause normally begins 8-10 years before menopause. It normally starts while you're in your mid-40s, although it might start in your 30s or earlier.

If you go through menopause before age 40, that's termed premature menopause. It may be caused by various medical disorders or treatments. If there is no medical or surgical explanation for early menopause, it's termed primary ovarian insufficiency. Early menopause may be caused by:

- Smoking or using other tobacco products.
- A family history of early menopause.
- A history of cancer therapy.
- Having your uterus or ovaries removed.

The usual period of perimenopause is roughly four years. Some individuals may only be in this stage for a few months, while others may be in this transition period for more than four years. If you've gone more than 12 months without having a period, you are no longer in perimenopause.

Navigating perimenopause might seem like going on an unfamiliar adventure, full of uncertainty, hardships, and times of deep growth. Yet, it's also a moment of empowerment and development — a chance to accept the changes occurring inside and retake control of one's health and vitality.

In this book, we'll go deep into the complexity of perimenopause, studying everything from the physiological changes happening in the body to practical solutions for managing symptoms and improving general well-being. This is aimed to equip you with the information, support, and empowerment you need to succeed during this shift.

How to Use This Book: A Step-by-Step Guide

Welcome to The Essential Guide to Perimenopause for Women Over 35! This comprehensive resource is meant to accompany you on your journey through perimenopause and offer you the information, methods, and resources you need to manage this transitional time with confidence and empowerment. Here's step-by-step guidance on how to get the most out of this book:

1. **Start with the Introduction:** Begin by reading the introduction to acquaint yourself with the objective of this book. Gain an idea of what to anticipate and how the information is arranged to take you through the many stages of perimenopause.

2. **Read Each Chapter Thoroughly:** Dive into each chapter, beginning with Chapter 1, and continue sequentially through the book. Each chapter discusses distinct subjects connected to perimenopause, from hormonal changes and symptoms to lifestyle measures and self-care practices.

3. **Take Notes and Reflect:** As you read, take notes on significant ideas, insights, and techniques that connect with you. Reflect on how the material pertains to your personal experiences and explore how you may

incorporate the advice and suggestions into your everyday life.

4. **Engage with Exercises and Activities:** Throughout the book, you'll discover exercises and activities meant to increase your learning and support personal development. Take the time to interact with these activities and reflect on your replies to acquire deeper insights into your health and well-being.

5. **Share Your Comment:** Your comment is crucial in creating future versions of this book and helping the author in addressing the needs and interests of readers. Share your ideas, opinions, and recommendations for improvement via reviews.

6. **Connect with the Author:** Connect with the author via her Author Central account to remain updated about forthcoming publications, unique material, and special deals. By following the author, you'll get rapid alerts whenever new articles are

produced, enabling you to remain involved and informed.

7. **Implement Actionable techniques:** Finally, take action on the techniques and advice presented in the book to promote your health and well-being throughout perimenopause. Experiment with multiple ways, measure your progress and adapt as required to discover what works best for you.

By following these steps and interacting actively with the material of this book, you'll be well-equipped to face the difficulties and possibilities of perimenopause with fortitude, grace, and empowerment. Here's to your path of discovery, development, and change!

Chapter 1: Hormones and Why They Are So Important

Hormones are sometimes referred to as the body's chemical messengers — complicated signalling molecules that play a critical role in regulating many physiological processes and sustaining general health and well-being. Produced by the endocrine glands and released into the circulation, hormones work as potent communicators, coordinating a broad variety of processes throughout the body.

Understanding hormones and their role in perimenopause is vital for navigating this shift with grace and resilience. Here's a full discussion of hormones and their role during perimenopause:

1. **Oestrogen:** Oestrogen is a major female sex hormone generated mostly by the ovaries, but minor quantities are also produced by the adrenal glands and fat cells. Oestrogen has a key function in regulating the menstrual cycle, supporting reproductive health, preserving bone density, and fostering good skin and hair. During perimenopause, oestrogen levels vary unexpectedly, resulting in irregular menstruation periods, hot flashes, vaginal dryness, and mood swings.

2. **Progesterone:** Progesterone is another key female sex hormone generated by the ovaries. It acts in concert with oestrogen to control the menstrual cycle and facilitate pregnancy. Progesterone helps thicken the uterine lining in preparation for implantation and supports pregnancy if conception occurs. During perimenopause, progesterone levels fall, resulting in irregular periods, mood swings, and changes in libido.

3. **Testosterone:** While commonly associated with males, testosterone is also found in women, albeit in lesser concentrations.

Testosterone has a function in preserving bone density, muscular mass, and libido, as well as promoting general energy and vitality. During perimenopause, testosterone levels may fall, leading to a loss in libido, diminished muscular mass, and exhaustion.

4. **Follicle-stimulating Hormone (FSH) and Luteinizing Hormone (LH):** FSH and LH are pituitary hormones that govern the menstrual cycle and ovulation. FSH encourages the development and maturity of ovarian follicles, whereas LH induces ovulation and the release of an egg from the ovary. During perimenopause, FSH and LH levels may rise as the ovaries become less sensitive to their signals, resulting in irregular menstruation periods and other symptoms.

5. **Cortisol:** Cortisol, frequently referred to as the "stress hormone," is generated by the adrenal glands in reaction to stress. Cortisol helps control metabolism, blood sugar levels, and the body's reaction to inflammation. During perimenopause, changes in oestrogen and progesterone levels might alter cortisol

production, thereby worsening stress and mood swings.

6. **Thyroid hormones:** Thyroid hormones, including thyroxine (T4) and triiodothyronine (T3), are generated by the thyroid gland and play a key role in regulating metabolism, energy generation, and body temperature. Thyroid function may be altered by hormonal changes during perimenopause, leading to symptoms such as tiredness, weight gain, and mood disorders.

Hormonal Regulation in Your Body

As much as 10-12 years before menopause, you might start to notice the consequences of minor hormonal changes beginning to develop. One of the most noticeable indicators is if you observe any variations in your menstrual periods. They may grow shorter, longer, or less regular in some manner.

Early in perimenopause, you may see a relative reduction in your progesterone levels, particularly if you "miss" ovulation in some cycles. Later in perimenopause, as you approach closer to running out of eggs and becoming menopausal, your oestrogen levels will also become substantially lower at times.

You have achieved menopause when you haven't ovulated for 12 months; that is, your ovaries have ceased generating eggs. Most women may notice this since their periods have ceased. Some may find it tougher to tell since they don't have periods. This may be related to a hysterectomy, endometrial ablation (to reduce heavy periods), or usage of hormone medications such as a Mirena IUD. Women who are taking the pill or other hormonal contraception that "induces" menstruation might be deceived into believing they're not menopausal.

During your reproductive years, ovaries cyclically generate oestrogen and progesterone. Once you stop ovulating at menopause, however, your oestrogen and progesterone levels are substantially lower.

Postmenopausally reproductive hormone levels are normally relatively low and steady. The mental instability and cyclical symptoms that women suffer in perimenopause may vanish again following menopause.

You may continue to suffer hot flushes for some time, however, as your body works to adapt to decreased oestrogen levels. One technique to treat hot flashes and nocturnal sweats is oestrogen therapy. This is a safe and extremely successful therapy choice for most women who are perimenopausal or recently menopausal.

Hormonal Fluctuations During Perimenopause

During perimenopause, women undergo severe hormonal swings as their bodies transition from the reproductive period to menopause. These oscillations are principally caused by changes in the function of the ovaries, which progressively reduce their production of oestrogen and progesterone. The hormonal changes that occur during perimenopause may vary greatly across people and may result in a variety of physical and mental problems. Here's a look at hormone variations during perimenopause:

1. **Oestrogen Fluctuations:** Oestrogen levels vary unpredictably during perimenopause, generally dropping steadily but occasionally

surging briefly. This hormonal instability may lead to irregular menstrual cycles, hot flashes, nocturnal sweats, vaginal dryness, mood swings, and changes in libido. Oestrogen is crucial for regulating the menstrual cycle, supporting reproductive health, preserving bone density, and fostering good skin and hair. As oestrogen levels fall during perimenopause, women may also suffer symptoms such as tiredness, joint discomfort, and trouble focusing.

2. **Progesterone Diminish:** Progesterone levels diminish during perimenopause as ovarian function declines. Progesterone is crucial for regulating the menstrual cycle, facilitating pregnancy, and maintaining general hormonal balance. The drop in progesterone levels may lead to irregular periods, mood swings, and changes in libido. Some women may also suffer symptoms such as anxiety, sleeplessness, and breast pain when progesterone levels decline.

3. **Follicle-Stimulating Hormone (FSH) Elevation:** FSH levels generally rise during

perimenopause as the body seeks to stimulate the ovaries to create more oestrogen. FSH is a pituitary hormone that plays a crucial function in the menstrual cycle by increasing the development and maturation of ovarian follicles. Elevated FSH levels are typically reported during perimenopause and are related to symptoms such as irregular menstruation periods and hot flashes.

4. **Luteinizing Hormone (LH) Fluctuations:** LH levels may also rise during perimenopause in response to decreased oestrogen levels. LH initiates ovulation, the release of an egg from the ovary, and stimulates the creation of progesterone by the corpus luteum. Fluctuations in LH levels may lead to irregular menstrual periods and other symptoms associated with perimenopause.

5. **Testosterone Fall:** Testosterone levels may fall gradually during perimenopause, but this hormone is predominantly related to men's health. Testosterone has a role in sustaining libido, muscular mass, and energy levels in women, as well as boosting general vitality

and well-being. As testosterone levels decline during perimenopause, women may suffer symptoms such as diminished libido, exhaustion, and changes in body composition.

6. **Other Hormonal Changes:** In addition to oestrogen, progesterone, FSH, LH, and testosterone, other hormones may also change during perimenopause. Cortisol, the "stress hormone," may be impacted by hormonal changes during perimenopause, thereby aggravating stress and mood swings. Thyroid hormones, which govern metabolism and energy production, may also be disrupted, leading to symptoms such as weariness, weight gain, and mood problems.

Impact of Hormonal Fluctuations on Menstrual Cycle and Symptoms

Every month throughout your reproductive years, your body prepares to prepare for a prospective pregnancy. Research reveals oestrogen, progesterone, testosterone, and your other female hormones all have a part in your monthly cycle.

First, your pituitary gland produces two hormones (FSH and LH) that go to your ovaries and indicate that it's time to release eggs. This causes your oestrogen levels to increase, and an egg is released.

Around this time, testosterone levels surge, enhancing your sex desire. After you ovulate, testosterone and oestrogen levels decline and your progesterone levels rise.

If you don't conceive, both oestrogen and progesterone decline. This might cause symptoms of PMS.

As you conclude your menstrual cycle, one of your progesterone hormones (prostaglandin) increases and stimulates uterine contractions. This causes the lining of your uterus to shed and you receive your period.

Imbalances in any of these essential hormones might alter your menstrual cycle and cause irregular periods and other symptoms connected to your reproductive cycle, including:

1. **Irregular Menstrual Periods:** One of the defining indications of perimenopause is irregularity in menstrual periods. Women may notice variations in the duration of their periods, unpredictability in the time of ovulation, and fluctuations in menstrual flow. Some cycles may be shorter or longer than typical, while others may be unusual in terms of timing or length. These anomalies are mostly due to variations in hormone levels, notably estrogen and progesterone, which drive the menstrual cycle.

2. **Changes in Menstrual Flow:** Perimenopause may also lead to changes in menstrual flow, including adjustments in the volume and length of bleeding. Some women may have larger or lighter periods than normal, while others may notice changes in the substance or color of menstrual blood. These alterations are generally ascribed to oscillations in hormone levels and changes in the uterine lining.

3. **Heavy or Prolonged Bleeding:** Some women may suffer periods of heavy or

prolonged bleeding during perimenopause, known as menorrhagia. This may be extremely disruptive and may result in exhaustion, anaemia, and other health difficulties. Menorrhagia is commonly caused by hormone imbalances, although other causes such as uterine fibroids or endometrial abnormalities may also contribute.

4. **Menstrual Cramps:** Some women may have increased menstrual cramps or pelvic pain during perimenopause. This may be related to variations in hormone levels, modifications in the uterine lining, or underlying problems like fibroids or endometriosis. Menstrual cramps may vary in strength and length and may be handled with over-the-counter pain medications, heat treatment, and relaxation methods.

5. **Mood Swings and Emotional Symptoms:** Hormonal variations during perimenopause may also impair mood and emotional well-being. Many women suffer mood swings, anger, anxiety, and despair at this period. These emotional symptoms may be

aggravated by other variables such as stress, sleep difficulties, and changes in lifestyle or relationships.

6. **Hot Flashes and Night Sweats:** Hot flashes and night sweats are frequent symptoms of perimenopause and are considered to be associated with variations in oestrogen levels. Hot flashes are characterised by abrupt sensations of warmth, flushing, and perspiration, typically accompanied by a fast pulse and palpitations. Night sweats are similar but occur during sleep and may interrupt sleep patterns and lead to exhaustion and daily sleepiness.

7. **Vaginal Dryness and Pain:** Declining oestrogen levels during perimenopause may contribute to vaginal dryness, itching, and pain. This may result in pain or discomfort during intercourse, urine symptoms such as urgency or frequency, and an increased risk of vaginal infections. Vaginal moisturisers, lubricants, and oestrogen treatment may help reduce these symptoms.

8. **Changes in Libido:** Many women report changes in libido or sexual drive during perimenopause. This might be attributed to hormonal swings, physical symptoms such as vaginal dryness or pain, or mental causes such as stress or relationship troubles. Open discussion with a spouse, therapy, and lifestyle modifications may help manage fluctuations in libido during perimenopause.

9. **Spotting or Breakthrough Bleeding:** Perimenopause may also be characterised by bouts of spotting or breakthrough bleeding between cycles. This may occur as a consequence of hormonal fluctuations, alterations in the uterine lining, or anomalies in ovulation. While spotting is normally not a reason for worry, it's crucial to visit a healthcare practitioner if it continues or is accompanied by other symptoms.

10. **Digestive Complaints, such as Constipation:** During perimenopause, hormone variations may affect several physical systems outside the reproductive and emotional domains. One area that is regularly

impacted, however seldom acknowledged, is the digestive system. Hormonal changes during perimenopause might alter gastrointestinal function, resulting in symptoms such as constipation

Imbalances may also create other concerns, such as difficulty sleeping, acne and skin complaints, problems with weight, and insulin resistance.

Chapter 2: Hormone Replacement Therapy (HRT)

Hormone replacement therapy (HRT) is a medication used to relieve menopausal symptoms. It replaces the hormones oestrogen and progesterone, which diminish to low levels as you approach menopause. Menopause symptoms HRT may help to treat include:

- Hot flushes
- Nocturnal sweats sleep troubles
- Mood swings
- Anxiety and poor mood vaginal dryness

Menopause is when your periods end owing to reduced hormone levels. It mainly affects women between the ages of 45 and 55 although it may develop younger. It affects anybody who has periods.

Oestrogen and progesterone are an integral feature of period cycles, ovulation, and pregnancy. They also maintain your bones healthy. As you become older, the loss of these hormones may have a huge influence on your health.

To replenish these hormones, you'll normally take a mix of oestrogen and progestogen. If you've undergone a hysterectomy to remove your womb you may take oestrogen on its own.

Who can take HRT?
You can normally take HRT if you're suffering from menopausal symptoms.

But HRT may not be appropriate if you:
- Have a history of breast cancer, ovarian cancer, or womb cancer.
- Have a history of blood clots – you may need to use patches or gels rather than pills.

- Having untreated high blood pressure – your blood pressure will need to be stabilised before you can start HRT.
- Have liver illness.
- Are pregnant – it's still possible to become pregnant while using HRT, therefore it's crucial to take contraception until 2 years following your last period if you're under 50, or for 1 year beyond the age of 50.

If any of these apply to you, alternatives to HRT may be considered instead.

Purpose and Benefits

Hormone Replacement Therapy (HRT) serves multiple objectives and provides different benefits for women suffering symptoms of hormonal imbalance, notably during menopause and perimenopause. Here are the primary uses and advantages of HRT:

1. **Alleviation of Menopausal Symptoms:** The main objective of HRT is to reduce the symptoms associated with menopause and perimenopause. These symptoms, including as hot flashes, night sweats, vaginal dryness,

mood swings, sleep difficulties, and cognitive impairments, are caused by falling levels of estrogen and progesterone in the body. HRT refills these hormone levels to ease symptoms and enhance overall quality of life.

2. **Relief from Vasomotor Symptoms:** Vasomotor symptoms, including hot flashes and night sweats, are among the most prevalent and annoying symptoms of menopause. HRT may give considerable relief from these symptoms by regulating hormone levels and lowering the frequency and intensity of hot flashes and night sweats. This may contribute to increased comfort, sleep quality, and everyday functioning for women suffering from these symptoms.

3. **Improvement of Vaginal Health:** Declining oestrogen levels after menopause may contribute to vaginal dryness, pain, and weakening of the vaginal tissues, known as vaginal atrophy. HRT may assist enhance vaginal health by restoring moisture, suppleness, and thickness to the vaginal tissues. This may ease symptoms such as

dryness, itching, burning, and discomfort during intercourse, boosting sexual enjoyment and closeness for women.

4. **Maintenance of Bone Health:** Oestrogen plays a critical function in maintaining bone density and preventing bone loss. Declining oestrogen levels following menopause raise the risk of osteoporosis, a disorder characterised by weaker bones and greater susceptibility to fractures. HRT may assist in preserving bone health by conserving bone density and lowering the incidence of osteoporosis and fractures, especially in women at greater risk.

5. **Protection of Cardiovascular Health:** Oestrogen has cardioprotective benefits, including lowering lipid profiles, decreasing inflammation, and boosting vascular health. Hormone Replacement Therapy may give cardiovascular advantages by improving lipid profiles, decreasing the risk of atherosclerosis, and lowering the risk of heart disease in certain women. However, the cardiovascular consequences of HRT may

vary based on variables such as age, medical history, and hormone dose.

6. **Enhancement of Cognitive Function:** Oestrogen may also have a role in cognitive function and brain health. Some study shows that HRT may have cognitive advantages, such as increasing memory, attention, and executive function, especially in women who undergo cognitive changes after menopause. However, further research is required to completely evaluate the effects of HRT on cognitive performance and dementia risk.

7. **Improvement of Mood and Emotional Well-being:** Hormonal variations during menopause may impair mood and emotional well-being, leading to symptoms such as mood swings, impatience, anxiety, and despair. HRT may help regulate hormone levels and alleviate mood symptoms in some women, boosting overall emotional well-being and quality of life.

8. **Reduction of Genitourinary Symptoms:** In addition to vaginal dryness and pain,

menopausal women may have urine symptoms such as urinary urgency, frequency, and incontinence. HRT may help ease these genitourinary symptoms by increasing vaginal health, lowering urinary tract infections, and strengthening bladder function.

9. **Maintenance of Skin Health:** Oestrogen has a role in maintaining skin moisture, suppleness, and collagen formation. Declining oestrogen levels during menopause may contribute to changes in skin texture, including dryness, thinning, and increased wrinkles. HRT may help improve skin health by restoring oestrogen levels, resulting in smoother, more youthful-looking skin and fewer indications of ageing.

10. **Reduction of Muscle and Joint Pain:** Hormonal imbalances during menopause might lead to muscle and joint pain, stiffness, and inflammation. Oestrogen has anti-inflammatory qualities and may help relieve pain and improve joint function in certain women. HRT may reduce muscle and

joint problems associated with menopause, boosting mobility and physical comfort.

11. **Prevention of Vaginal and Urinary Tract Infections:** Vaginal atrophy, marked by thinning and drying of the vaginal tissues, may increase the risk of vaginal infections, such as yeast infections and bacterial vaginosis. HRT may help restore vaginal health by increasing moisture and acidity in the vaginal environment, lowering the incidence of infections. Additionally, HRT may help prevent urinary tract infections by increasing bladder function and lowering urinary symptoms.

12. **Enhancement of Sexual Function and Pleasure:** Hormonal changes during menopause may impact sexual desire, arousal, and pleasure for many women. Vaginal dryness, pain, and changes in desire may significantly impair sexual function and intimacy. HRT may assist improve sexual health by treating vaginal dryness, improving desire, and promoting sexual pleasure. This may lead to enhanced sexual interactions and

general quality of life for women and their partners.

13. **Management of Menopausal Symptoms in Breast Cancer Survivors:** Women who have had treatment for breast cancer may suffer menopausal symptoms as a consequence of chemotherapy, radiation therapy, or hormone therapy. HRT may be investigated as a therapy option for controlling menopausal symptoms in breast cancer survivors, especially for those with severe symptoms that adversely influence quality of life. However, the use of HRT in breast cancer survivors must be carefully examined and individualised depending on the kind and stage of the disease, treatment history, and risk factors.

14. **Prevention of Colorectal Cancer:** Some studies show that HRT may have a preventive effect against colorectal cancer, especially in postmenopausal women. Oestrogen may exhibit anticancer actions on the colon by lowering inflammation, slowing cell growth, and increasing apoptosis (cell death) in

colorectal cancer cells. However, additional study is required to establish the function of HRT in colorectal cancer prevention and to discover the appropriate duration and dose of hormone treatment for this purpose.

Dosage & Administration

This might vary based on variables such as the kind of hormones used, the formulation of the medicine, the individual's medical history, and the degree of menopausal symptoms. HRT should always be administered and managed by a healthcare practitioner to ensure safety and effectiveness. Here's a full review of the dose and administration of HRT:

1. **Initial Assessment and Assessment:** Before commencing HRT, a full medical assessment is important to analyse the individual's general health, medical history, risk factors, and menopausal symptoms. This evaluation may involve a physical examination, review of medical history, assessment of symptoms, and laboratory testing to detect hormone levels and screen for underlying health issues.

2. **Selection of Hormone Therapy:** Based on the individual's medical history, symptoms, and treatment objectives, the healthcare professional will identify the most suitable kind of hormone therapy and formulation. HRT may entail the use of oestrogen alone (for women who have had a hysterectomy) or a combination of oestrogen and progesterone (for women with an intact uterus). The choice of hormone treatment may also rely on variables such as the woman's age, menopausal state, and risk factors for specific health issues.

3. **Dosage and Formulation:** Hormone Replacement Therapy is available in different forms and dosages, including oral pills, transdermal patches, creams, gels, sprays, and vaginal preparations. The dose and formulation of HRT will be tailored depending on parameters such as the severity of symptoms, hormone levels, responsiveness to therapy, and personal preferences. The healthcare professional will prescribe the lowest effective dosage of hormones for the

shortest term required to meet treatment objectives and limit the risk of unwanted effects.

4. **Titration of Dose:** In certain situations, the dose of HRT may need to be modified over time depending on the individual's reaction to therapy and changes in symptoms. The healthcare professional may titrate the dose of hormones up or down as required to obtain maximum symptom alleviation while minimising adverse effects. Regular follow-up sessions are required to assess the individual's development and change therapy as appropriate.

5. **Administration Instructions:** The administration instructions for HRT will vary on the individual formulation recommended. Oral pills are normally taken once a day with or without meals, ideally at the same time each day. Transdermal patches are applied to clean, dry skin on the belly, buttocks, or thighs and are changed according to the suggested schedule (e.g., weekly or twice weekly). Topical creams, gels, and sprays are

applied to the skin as indicated, generally once or twice daily. Vaginal preparations, such as lotions, pills, or rings, are put into the vagina as instructed, often on a daily or weekly basis.

6. **Monitoring and Follow-up:** Regular monitoring and follow-up sessions are required for persons undergoing HRT to assess therapy effectiveness, check hormone levels, and evaluate for any side effects or problems. The healthcare practitioner will examine symptoms, do physical exams, and request laboratory testing as required to confirm the safety and efficacy of HRT. Adjustments to dose or treatment regimen may be changed depending on the individual's reaction to therapy and changes in health condition over time.

7. **Duration of Treatment:** The duration of Hormone Replacement Therapy will vary based on variables such as the individual's age, menopausal state, symptom intensity, and treatment objectives. In general, HRT is prescribed for the shortest term required to

treat menopausal symptoms and enhance quality of life. The healthcare practitioner will regularly examine the necessity for continuing therapy and discuss alternatives for termination or tapering of HRT depending on the individual's preferences and risk factors.

8. **Discontinuation of Treatment:** When terminating Hormone Replacement Therapy, it is advisable to gently reduce the dose rather than stopping suddenly to avoid the risk of rebound symptoms and withdrawal effects. The healthcare practitioner will give advise on how to properly withdraw HRT and may propose other medication choices or lifestyle adjustments to manage menopausal symptoms following cessation.

Types of Hormones Used in HRT

The kinds of hormones used in HRT might vary based on various aspects but the ultimate objective entails the supplementing of hormones to reduce symptoms linked with hormonal imbalances such as the individual's medical history, symptoms, and treatment goals. Here are the kinds of hormones widely used in HRT:

1. **Oestrogen:** Oestrogen is the key female sex hormone important for regulating several biological processes, including reproductive health, bone density, cardiovascular health, and cognitive function. During menopause and perimenopause, oestrogen levels fall, leading to symptoms such as hot flashes, vaginal dryness, mood changes, and bone loss. Oestrogen replacement treatment is the cornerstone of HRT and tries to restore oestrogen levels to reduce these symptoms and promote general well-being.

   Types of Oestrogen: There are various kinds of oestrogen used in HRT, including:
   - **Estradiol:** This is the most powerful and physiologically active type of oestrogen and is regarded as the ideal form of oestrogen replacement treatment. Estradiol may be taken orally, transdermally (by patches, gels, or creams), intramuscularly, or vaginally.

- **Conjugated Equine Estrogens (CEEs):** These are generated from the urine of pregnant mares and include a combination of estrogens, including estrone sulphate, equilin sulphate, and equilin. CEEs are accessible in oral tablet form and are less widely utilised than estradiol.

- **Estropipate:** This synthetic oestrogen is manufactured from estrone and is accessible in oral tablet form. Estropipate is less effective than estradiol but is occasionally preferable for women who cannot handle other types of oestrogen.

2. **Progesterone:** Progesterone is another key female sex hormone that works in concert with oestrogen to control the menstrual cycle and maintain reproductive health. In women with an intact uterus, progesterone is important to preserve the uterine lining (endometrium) from overgrowth and lower the risk of endometrial hyperplasia or cancer. Progesterone replacement treatment is generally paired with oestrogen therapy in

women with an intact uterus to offer full hormone replacement and limit the risk of endometrial problems.

Types of Progesterone: Progesterone used in HRT may be taken from natural sources (bioidentical progesterone) or produced in a laboratory (progestins).

- **Bioidentical progesterone:** Is structurally identical to the progesterone generated by the ovaries and is regarded as the ideal type of progesterone replacement treatment.
- **Progestins:** Are synthetic substances that imitate the actions of progesterone but may have variable pharmacological characteristics and negative effect profiles.

3. **Testosterone:** Testosterone is often thought to be the male sex hormone, but it also plays a critical role in women's health, including sexual function, desire, muscle mass, bone density, and mood control. Testosterone levels fall with age, especially during and after menopause, resulting in symptoms such

as lower libido, weariness, physical weakness, and mood disorders. Testosterone replacement treatment may be administered as part of HRT to address these symptoms and enhance general well-being in women with low testosterone levels.

Types of Testosterone: Testosterone replacement treatment for women often includes the use of transdermal testosterone formulations, such as patches, gels, or creams. These formulations are applied to the skin and give a regulated amount of testosterone into the circulation. Oral testosterone treatment is not routinely utilised in women owing to the risk of liver damage and other adverse effects.

4. **DHEA (Dehydroepiandrosterone):** DHEA is a precursor hormone that is transformed into oestrogen and testosterone in the body. DHEA levels diminish with age, and supplementation with DHEA may be explored as part of HRT to treat symptoms such as tiredness, mood changes, and lower libido. However, the use of DHEA in HRT is

less prevalent than oestrogen, progesterone, and testosterone replacement treatment, and its effectiveness and safety in women need additional investigation.

5. **Bioidentical Hormones:** Bioidentical hormones are hormones that are structurally identical to those generated by the human body. Bioidentical hormones are frequently obtained from plant sources (such as soy or yam) and are compounded into tailored formulations depending on the individual's exact hormone levels and treatment requirements. Bioidentical hormone therapy (also known as bioidentical hormone replacement therapy or BHRT) is frequently used as an alternative to traditional HRT, especially for women who want natural or personalised treatment alternatives.

Methods of Administration

Methods of administration relate to the numerous methods by which Hormone Replacement Therapy (HRT) drugs are administered into the body. The choice of delivery technique relies on aspects such as the kind of hormones used, individual preferences, convenience, and treatment objectives. Here are several ways of administration for HRT:

1. **Oral Tablets:** Oral tablets are one of the most frequent and convenient means of taking HRT drugs. Oestrogen, progesterone, and combination hormone therapy are available in oral tablet form and are normally taken once a day with or without meals. Oral pills are simple to take and give a regular amount of hormones, making them acceptable for many women. However, oral tablets may be linked with gastrointestinal side effects such as nausea, bloating, and indigestion, and may need frequent liver function monitoring in certain individuals.

2. **Transdermal Patches:** Transdermal patches are adhesive patches that transfer hormones via the skin and into the circulation. Oestrogen and combination hormone therapy are available in transdermal patch form and are placed to clean, dry skin on the belly, buttocks, or thighs. Transdermal patches allow a continuous, regulated release of

hormones over a specific time (e.g., 3-7 days) and provide benefits such as avoidance of first-pass metabolism in the liver and decreased risk of gastrointestinal adverse effects. However, some women may have skin irritation or allergic responses at the patch location.

3. **Topical Creams, Gels, and Sprays:** Topical formulations of hormones, such as creams, gels, and sprays, are applied directly to the skin and absorbed into the circulation. Oestrogen, progesterone, and testosterone treatments are available in topical formulations and are commonly applied to clean, dry skin on locations such as the inner arms, thighs, belly, or chest. Topical formulations give flexibility in dosage and enable tailored therapy depending on the woman's requirements and preferences. However, absorption may vary based on variables such as skin thickness, moisture, and application method.

4. **Vaginal Preparations:** Vaginal preparations are especially intended for local delivery to

the vaginal tissues and are used to treat symptoms such as vaginal dryness, pain, and urinary symptoms. Oestrogen treatment is offered in several vaginal forms, including creams, pills, rings, and suppositories. Vaginal preparations distribute hormones directly to the vaginal tissues, where they may give focused relief from symptoms with low systemic absorption. However, vaginal preparations may be linked with local side effects such as vaginal discomfort, discharge, or spotting.

5. **Injections:** Injections are another means of giving hormones for HRT, especially testosterone treatment. Testosterone injections are commonly delivered intramuscularly (into the muscle) or subcutaneously (under the skin) and offer a regulated amount of hormone straight into the circulation. Testosterone injections may be delivered at home or in a healthcare environment, depending on the individual's preferences and healthcare provider's recommendations. However, injections may

be accompanied by pain at the injection site and need frequent delivery intervals.

6. **Implants:** Hormone implants are tiny, flexible devices that are inserted beneath the skin and deliver hormones slowly over a lengthy time. Testosterone implants are offered for testosterone replacement treatment and are implanted into the adipose tissue of the buttocks or belly. Hormone implants give long-lasting symptom alleviation and remove the requirement for daily dosage or frequent delivery. However, implantation needs a small surgical procedure and may be linked with hazards such as infection, migration, or scarring at the implant site.

7. **Sublingual Tablets or Troches:** Sublingual tablets or troches are inserted beneath the tongue and allowed to dissolve, allowing for quick absorption of hormones into the circulation. Oestrogen and progesterone medications are available in sublingual formulations and provide benefits such as avoiding first-pass metabolism in the liver

and enabling fast beginning of action. Sublingual administration may be chosen by women who have difficulties swallowing oral pills or who want a non-invasive mode of delivery.

Hormone replacements aren't a one-shot drug for a specific ailment, but a therapy plan that may endure for the length of a person's life. It's crucial to select the drug and delivery method that matches each patient best so that their therapy is as comfortable as possible.

Even if the variety seems a little perplexing at first, your clinician will be there to guide you through the advantages and drawbacks of each choice and how it may fit. There's an excellent selection for anybody who needs it, no matter their lifestyle, medical, or economic circumstances.

Side Effects and Associated Risks

Side effects are possible unpleasant responses or unforeseen outcomes that may arise as a result of Hormone Replacement Therapy (HRT). While HRT may successfully reduce menopausal symptoms and enhance the quality of life for many women, it is vital to be informed of the possible adverse effects associated with hormone treatment. Here are typical adverse effects related to HRT:

1. **Breast Discomfort or Swelling:** HRT, especially oestrogen treatment, may induce breast discomfort, swelling, or enlargement in some women. These breast alterations are generally transient and may resolve with ongoing therapy or modification of hormone dose. However, breast discomfort or swelling should be quickly reported to a healthcare physician for further assessment, as it may suggest underlying hormonal imbalance or breast health issues.

2. **Nausea and Gastrointestinal Upset:** Oral oestrogen medication, in particular, may be accompanied by gastrointestinal side effects such as nausea, bloating, indigestion, or stomach pain. These symptoms are normally moderate and fleeting, but if they continue or become troublesome, the healthcare practitioner may consider taking hormone medicine with meals or switching to a new

formulation or method of administration to avoid gastrointestinal discomfort.

3. **Headaches:** Some women may develop headaches or migraines as a side effect of HRT, especially during the beginning phases of therapy or with changes in hormone dose. Hormonal variations may influence blood vessel dilatation and neurotransmitter levels in the brain, thereby inducing headaches or migraines in vulnerable people. Headaches related to HRT are generally mild to moderate in intensity and may improve with time or with modifications to hormone treatment.

4. **Fluid Retention and Bloating:** Oestrogen medication, particularly at higher dosages, may induce fluid retention and bloating in some women. Fluid retention may contribute to edema or puffiness in the hands, feet, ankles, or cheeks, and may worsen symptoms such as breast tenderness or pain. Maintaining a balanced diet, staying hydrated, and participating in regular physical exercise might help minimise fluid

retention and relieve bloating associated with HRT.

5. **Mood Changes and Emotional Symptoms:** Hormonal variations during menopause and HRT may impair mood and emotional well-being, leading to symptoms such as mood swings, impatience, anxiety, or despair. While HRT may reduce mood issues in many women, some people may suffer worsening mood or emotional symptoms as a side effect of hormone treatment. It is vital to monitor mood changes attentively and get help from a healthcare practitioner or mental health professional if required.

6. **Vaginal Bleeding or Spotting:** Women using oestrogen and progesterone combination therapy may have vaginal bleeding or spotting, especially during the first few months of treatment or with changes in hormone dose. Hormone treatment may disrupt the uterine lining (endometrium) and menstrual cycle, leading to irregular bleeding patterns or breakthrough bleeding. Vaginal bleeding or spotting should be quickly

checked by a healthcare practitioner to rule out underlying gynaecological disorders or endometrial abnormalities.

7. **Changes in Libido and Sexual Function:** Hormonal changes during menopause and HRT may impair libido (sex desire) and sexual function in certain women. While HRT may relieve vaginal dryness, pain, and libido in many persons, other women may suffer changes in sexual desire, arousal, or pleasure as a side effect of hormone treatment. Open discussion with a partner and healthcare practitioner, as well as the study of alternate treatment options or treatments, may assist in resolving sexual problems linked with HRT.

8. **Changes in Weight or Body Composition:** Hormonal variations during menopause and HRT may impact weight management and body composition in certain women. Oestrogen treatment, in particular, may impact fat distribution, metabolism, and appetite management, possibly resulting in changes in body weight or shape. Regular

physical exercise, appropriate eating habits, and lifestyle alterations may help minimise changes in weight or body composition related to HRT and enhance general health and well-being.

9. **Increased Risk of Blood Clots:** Oestrogen medication, particularly when taken in higher dosages or conjunction with progestins, may raise the risk of blood clots (venous thromboembolism) in certain women. Blood clots may form in the deep veins of the legs (deep vein thrombosis) or migrate to the lungs (pulmonary embolism), leading to potentially fatal problems. Women with a history of blood clots, cardiovascular illness, or risk factors for thromboembolism should explore the possible risks and benefits of HRT with their healthcare practitioner and consider alternate treatment options.

10. **Breast Cancer Risk:** Hormone Replacement Therapy has been connected with a slightly increased risk of breast cancer, especially with long-term usage or specific hormone formulations. Oestrogen medication,

particularly when paired with progestins, may enhance cell growth and proliferation in the breast tissue, thus raising the risk of breast cancer development. Women contemplating HRT should examine their unique breast cancer risk factors with their healthcare practitioner and assess the possible hazards and benefits of hormone therapy based on their particular medical history and treatment objectives.

11. **Endometrial Cancer Risk:** Oestrogen treatment without progesterone supplementation (in women with an intact uterus) may raise the risk of endometrial cancer (cancer of the lining of the uterus) owing to unopposed oestrogen stimulation of the endometrial tissue. Progesterone has a protective function in the uterus by countering the effects of oestrogen and lowering the chance of endometrial hyperplasia or cancer. Women contemplating oestrogen therapy should explore the inclusion of progesterone or alternate treatment options with their healthcare

physicians to decrease the risk of endometrial cancer.

12. **Cardiovascular Concerns:** Hormone Replacement Therapy has been connected with possible cardiovascular concerns, including an increased risk of stroke, heart attack, or cardiovascular events in certain women. Oestrogen treatment may have both favourable and detrimental effects on cardiovascular health, depending on variables such as the woman's age, menopausal state, underlying health issues, and hormone formulation. Women with pre-existing cardiovascular illness, risk factors for heart disease, or a history of thromboembolic events should address the possible cardiovascular hazards of HRT with their healthcare practitioner and explore alternate treatment options.

13. **Gallbladder Disease:** Oestrogen medication, especially oral oestrogen, may raise the risk of gallbladder disease, such as gallstones, in certain women. Oestrogen may influence bile composition and gallbladder function,

perhaps leading to the production of gallstones or gallbladder inflammation. Women with a history of gallbladder disease or risk factors for gallstones should discuss the possible dangers of HRT with their healthcare professionals and seek alternate treatment options.

Alternative Therapies and Non-Hormonal Options

Alternative treatments and non-hormonal methods for treating menopausal symptoms give women extra choices for symptom alleviation and general well-being. These treatments concentrate on resolving menopausal symptoms with lifestyle adjustments, dietary changes, herbal supplements, and mind-body practices. While they may not be as powerful as Hormone Replacement Therapy (HRT), many women find alternative treatments to be successful in lowering symptoms and enhancing quality of life.

1. **Lifestyle Modifications**
   - **Regular Exercise:** Engaging in regular physical exercise, such as

walking, swimming, or yoga, may help decrease menopausal symptoms, including hot flashes, mood swings, and sleep difficulties. Exercise also increases general health, cardiovascular fitness, and bone density.

- **Healthy Diet:** Adopting a balanced diet rich in fruits, vegetables, whole grains, and lean meats may help promote hormonal balance, control weight, and lower the risk of chronic illnesses. Some women find that avoiding particular triggers, like spicy foods, caffeine, and alcohol, may help lessen hot flashes and other symptoms.

- **Stress Management:** Practising stress-reducing strategies, such as mindfulness meditation, deep breathing exercises, or progressive muscle relaxation, may help decrease anxiety, improve mood, and promote general well-being throughout menopause.

2. Herbal Supplements

- **Black Cohosh:** Black cohosh is a botanical supplement obtained from the roots of the Actaea racemosa plant. It is often used to relieve menopausal symptoms, including hot flashes, nocturnal sweats, and mood swings. While the specific mechanism of action is not entirely known, some research shows that black cohosh may function as a phytoestrogen and interact with serotonin receptors in the brain.

- **Soy Isoflavones:** Soy isoflavones are plant-based chemicals found in soybeans and soy products. They have modest oestrogen-like actions in the body and may help decrease menopausal symptoms, such as hot flashes and vaginal dryness. Soy isoflavones are available as dietary supplements and may be especially effective for women who choose natural or non-hormonal choices for symptom alleviation.

- **Red Clover:** Red clover is another source of phytoestrogens, including genistein and daidzein, which may help ease menopausal symptoms. Red clover supplements are available in numerous forms, including capsules, pills, and teas, and are widely used to alleviate hot flashes, night sweats, and mood swings.

- **Dong Quai:** Dong Quai, also known as Angelica sinensis, is a plant extensively used in traditional Chinese medicine to treat gynaecological disorders, including menopausal symptoms. It is considered to have estrogenic actions and may help manage hormonal balance, minimise hot flashes, and promote general well-being.

3. Acupuncture: Acupuncture is a traditional Chinese medical treatment that includes the insertion of tiny needles into particular places on the body to enhance energy flow and aid healing. Some women found acupuncture to be beneficial in relieving menopausal symptoms, including hot flashes, night sweats, sleeplessness, and mood changes. While the mechanisms of effect are not entirely understood, acupuncture may modify hormone levels, increase blood flow, and boost neurotransmitter activity in the brain.

4. Mind-Body Techniques

- **Yoga:** Yoga combines physical postures, breathing exercises, and meditation to improve relaxation, flexibility, and awareness. Some women find that doing yoga frequently may help decrease stress, enhance sleep quality, and relieve menopausal symptoms, such as hot flashes, mood swings, and lethargy.

- **Meditation and Mindfulness:** Mindfulness meditation entails concentrating on the present moment and fostering awareness of thoughts, emotions, and body sensations without judgement. Regular meditation practice may help decrease stress, anxiety, and depressive symptoms, and enhance general emotional well-being throughout menopause.

- **Biofeedback:** Biofeedback is a method that teaches people to manage physiological reactions, such as heart rate, blood pressure, and muscular tension, via self-regulation and feedback. Biofeedback training may help women manage symptoms such as hot flashes, night sweats, and tension by increasing relaxation and stress reduction.

5. Vaginal Moisturisers and Lubricants: For women suffering vaginal dryness, discomfort, or painful intercourse, over-the-counter vaginal moisturisers and lubricants may give relief. These products assist moisturise the vaginal tissues, minimise friction during intercourse, and increase overall comfort and sexual pleasure. Vaginal moisturisers are often used daily to preserve vaginal moisture and suppleness, whereas lubricants are used as required before sexual activity.

6. Selective Serotonin Reuptake Inhibitors (SSRIs) and Selective Serotonin-Norepinephrine Reuptake Inhibitors (SNRIs): Some antidepressant drugs, such as SSRIs (e.g., paroxetine, fluoxetine) and SNRIs (e.g., venlafaxine, duloxetine), have been proven to lower the frequency and intensity of hot flashes in menopausal women. While the specific mechanism of action is not entirely known, these drugs may modify neurotransmitter levels in the brain and assist in the control of thermoregulatory systems involved in hot flash development.

Chapter 3: Progesterone Intolerance and Oestrogen Dominance

Understanding progesterone intolerance and oestrogen dominance is vital for women navigating the intricacies of hormonal swings during perimenopause. These diseases may profoundly impair a woman's health and well-being, resulting in a range of symptoms and serious health repercussions.

Progesterone Intolerance: Progesterone intolerance occurs when the body has trouble tolerating or metabolising progesterone, a hormone necessary for reproductive health and menstrual cycle management. Progesterone prepares the uterine lining for future pregnancy, maintains pregnancy, and helps regulate the menstrual cycle. However, some women may develop harmful effects from progesterone exposure.

Women who are particularly sensitive to progesterone might have major premenstrual symptoms such as premenstrual syndrome (PMS), premenstrual aggravation of existing symptoms (PME), or premenstrual depression or premenstrual dysphoric disorder (PMDD).

Causes and Symptoms

What Causes Progesterone Intolerance?
The specific aetiology of progesterone intolerance is not entirely known. It may be altered by things such as:
- Hormone imbalances
- Genetic predisposition
- Sensitivity to progesterone receptors
- Underlying health conditions

Symptoms of Progesterone Intolerance
Progesterone intolerance may show via a multitude of symptoms. They may vary amongst persons, in

intensity, length, and kinds. Let's look at the following symptoms:

1. **Physical Symptoms:** The physical symptoms of progesterone intolerance might include:
   - **Mood Swings and irritation:** Some people may suffer mood variations, ranging from moderate irritation to more dramatic mood swings.
   - **Fatigue and Drowsiness:** Because progesterone is converted to allopregnanolone in the brain (a relaxing neurosteroid), it helps promote sleep and should be administered before going to bed. For women with heightened sensitivity to this, it might create an excessive sensation of tiredness or lethargy.
   - **Breast soreness:** Increased progesterone levels may contribute to breast soreness or sensitivity.
   - **Headaches or Migraines:** Some persons may be more prone to headaches or migraines in reaction to high progesterone.

- **Digestive Discomfort:** Progesterone has a calming impact on the body. Relaxing the stomach might impede digestion, perhaps leading to symptoms like bloating, constipation, or diarrhoea.
- **Fluid Retention:** Swelling or bloating, especially in the extremities, may develop with progesterone intolerance.
- **Skin Rashes:** Some women experience another form of response with progesterone use: autoimmune progesterone dermatitis. These ladies get a rash after exposure to progesterone/progestogens.

It occurs in a rash in the luteal phase of the menstrual cycle (1-2 weeks before the period begins) or while taking progesterone as a hormone therapy.

2. Psychological Symptoms: In addition to physical symptoms, progesterone intolerance may also produce psychological difficulties. These may include:

- **Anxiety:** Elevated levels of progesterone might produce anxiety in certain persons who are sensitive to its effects.
- **Depression:** Progesterone is known to alter neurotransmitters and mood control in the brain. For individuals with greater sensitivity.

3. Metabolic Symptoms: Progesterone resistance might also appear via metabolic symptoms. These may include:

- **Weight Gain:** Elevated progesterone levels may occasionally contribute to increased water retention and bloating, leading to temporary weight gain.
- **Insulin Resistance:** Some patients with progesterone intolerance may develop increased insulin resistance, which may influence blood sugar levels and raise cholesterol levels.

Oestrogen dominance: Oestrogen and progesterone work effectively together to prevent the lining of your uterus from being overly thick. Some people's bodies don't create enough progesterone, resulting in what's called unopposed oestrogen. Unopposed oestrogen is termed oestrogen dominance in certain medical literature. Without progesterone's balancing action, oestrogen may work overtime in your body and create cell overgrowth, such as tumours in your uterine lining.

How does excessive oestrogen affect your body as a woman? It's unusual for your levels to be high due to the oestrogen you're making. It's more probable that your oestrogen levels are elevated because of the drugs you're taking. For instance, you may experience a decreased sex desire due to high oestrogen levels, but this is most likely caused by your birth control tablets – not your body's natural oestrogen.

Elevated oestrogen unrelated to medication is most likely caused by PCOS before menopause. After menopause, high levels are more prevalent if you are overweight/obese.

If you're a trans guy or nonbinary person with a vagina, excessive oestrogen levels may hinder your body from having the outward look you'd prefer. If this is the case, masculinizing hormone treatment may be a possibility for you. This therapy entails taking testosterone to acquire secondary sex characteristics including increased muscle mass and facial and body hair.

What causes high oestrogen levels? Your oestrogen levels may be elevated because:
- Your body is creating too much oestrogen.
- You're receiving too much oestrogen in the medication you're taking.
- Your body's not breaking down oestrogen and eliminating it from your body as it should.

A multitude of causes may lead to excessive oestrogen, including:
- **Medications:** Hormone treatment to raise low oestrogen levels may cause your levels to become excessively high initially. It may take some time to get the dose perfect. (high-dose oral contraceptives/birth control tablets).
- **Body fat:** Fat tissue (adipose tissue) secretes oestrogen. Having a high amount of body fat might contribute to elevated oestrogen levels.
- **Stress:** Your body generates the hormone cortisol in reaction to stress. Producing large

quantities of cortisol in reaction to stress might reduce your body's capacity to generate progesterone. The oestrogen in your body is left uncontrolled by progesterone.

- **Alcohol:** Drinking too much alcohol might boost your oestrogen levels and limit your body's capacity to break down (metabolise) oestrogen.

- **Liver problems:** Your liver breaks down oestrogen and removes it from your body. If your liver's not working appropriately, too much oestrogen may build. Too few digestive enzymes, too much nasty gut flora (dysbiosis), insufficient magnesium levels, and too little fibre in your diet might inhibit your liver from eliminating excess oestrogen.

- **Synthetic xenoestrogens:** Synthetic xenoestrogens are substances prevalent in the environment that function like oestrogen once they're inside your body. They may raise your oestrogen levels. Xenoestrogens include bisphenol A (BPA) and phthalates. Both of these compounds are utilised in different polymers. Xenoestrogens may also be discovered in insecticides, home cleaning goods, and certain soaps and shampoos.

Strategies for Managing Hormonal Imbalances

Understanding progesterone intolerance and oestrogen dominance is critical for women navigating the intricacies of hormonal swings throughout perimenopause and beyond. These diseases indicate abnormalities in important reproductive hormones that may impair numerous areas of health and well-being.

Managing Progesterone Intolerance

1. **Check in with your Healthcare Provider:** If you encounter signs of progesterone intolerance, speak to your healthcare professional. They might examine your therapy and propose different choices.

2. **Alternative Progesterone Formulations:** Women with progesterone intolerance from synthetic progestins/progestogens may tolerate natural progesterone better (such as micronised progesterone/ Utrogestan/ Prometrium).

3. **Alternate Progesterone Delivery Methods:** Some women who have problems with progesterone intolerance orally do tolerate progesterone administered via different routes.

   A Mirena coil (IUD) releases levonorgestrel in low dosage locally into the uterus.

   Utrogestan or Prometrium (body-similar natural progesterone) may be used off-licence as vaginal progesterone pessaries, providing the progesterone directly where it's required and having fewer system effects.

   In other places like Australia, you may take a combination of oestrogen and progestogen patch (Estalis) therefore this may also have lower side effects.

   As none of these techniques are oral, they are frequently linked with a lesser incidence of progesterone intolerance.

4. **Reduce Progesterone Dose:** Using a lower dosage of oestrogen and progesterone may provide you with the advantages of HRT with fewer side effects of progesterone intolerance.

5. **Non-hormonal therapy for menopause:** Some ladies want to quit progesterone usage completely. They may utilise various medications such as antidepressants, clonidine, gabapentin. Also, vaginal oestrogen may be utilised without the requirement for progesterone.

6. **Surgical Alternatives:** Where other treatments are not beneficial, a hysterectomy would mean you can continue to take oestrogen without the need to use progesterone. However, all operations including a hysterectomy come with their dangers so make sure you get all your concerns addressed about this with your gynaecologist.

7. **Monitoring and Communication:** Tracking your symptoms helps your health professional assist you in making the best choices about your symptoms and your hormone therapy. Let your healthcare provider know if you have problems with your treatment.

Managing Oestrogen Dominance

The therapies your practitioner offers will depend on what's causing your elevated oestrogen levels. In certain circumstances, lifestyle adjustments may assist. If high oestrogen levels raise your cancer risk or exacerbate the cancer you already have, your physician may suggest more aggressive therapies.

There are few drugs that directly lower oestrogen. Usually, what's required is to discover the underlying problem and address this first.

1. **Lifestyle:** Making certain lifestyle modifications may help reduce your oestrogen levels. Your provider may propose that you:

2. **Decrease your proportion of body fat:** Decreasing your body fat may lessen the quantity of oestrogen that your fat cells release. Talk to your provider or a nutrition consultant about ways to safely lower your proportion of body fat so that you're obtaining the nutrients you need.

3. **Relieve Stress:** Decreasing the amount of stress hormones your body generates may help keep your oestrogen and progesterone levels balanced.

4. **Eat a nutritious diet:** Eating a low-fat, high-fibre diet with very little processed sugar will make it simpler for your liver to metabolise oestrogen.

5. **Limit your alcohol intake:** Eliminating alcohol or drinking in moderation might assist your liver break down oestrogen.

6. **Reduce your exposure to synthetic xenoestrogens:** It's hard to avoid synthetic xenoestrogens altogether, but you can minimise your exposure. Avoid pesticides that contain xenoestrogens by selecting all-natural organic foods and eating hormone-free meat products. Purchase things in steel and glass containers instead of plastic ones when you can.

7. **Liver Support:** Support liver health and detoxification processes with dietary

interventions, such as ingesting foods high in antioxidants (e.g., berries, leafy greens, turmeric), and avoiding excessive alcohol intake.

Chapter 4: Thyroid Health and Perimenopause

As women move through perimenopause, a time defined by hormonal swings and changes, they may confront different transformations in their general health and well-being. One key factor frequently disregarded is thyroid health. The thyroid gland plays a critical role in controlling metabolism, energy levels, mood, and general hormonal balance. However, thyroid dysfunction may frequently coincide with the start of perimenopause, leading to a plethora of symptoms that might mimic or intensify those linked with hormonal shifts. In this chapter, we will dig into the delicate link between thyroid health and perimenopause, studying the possible implications of thyroid dysfunction on women's health during this transitional era of life. By understanding the connection between thyroid function and perimenopause, women may make proactive efforts to promote their thyroid health and maximise overall well-being during this transitional time of life.

Hypothyroidism in Middle-Aged Women

Hypothyroidism is a common endocrine condition marked by an underactive thyroid gland, resulting in inadequate synthesis of thyroid hormones. Middle-aged women are especially sensitive to hypothyroidism, and its incidence tends to grow with age. Understanding the origins, symptoms, diagnosis, and treatment of hypothyroidism in middle-aged women is critical for delivering appropriate healthcare during this period of life.

Thyroid Function and Regulation: The thyroid gland, placed in the neck, generates thyroid hormones - thyroxine (T4) and triiodothyronine (T3) - crucial for regulating metabolism, energy generation, body temperature, and other physiological functions. Thyroid function is controlled by the hypothalamic-pituitary-thyroid (HPT) axis. The hypothalamus secretes thyrotropin-releasing hormone (TRH), causing the pituitary gland to produce thyroid-stimulating hormone (TSH). TSH then induces the thyroid gland to create and release thyroid hormones. Optimal thyroid function relies on the complex balance of this feedback mechanism.

Causes of Hypothyroidism

1. **Autoimmune Thyroiditis:** Hashimoto's thyroiditis is the most prevalent cause of hypothyroidism in middle-aged women. It happens when the immune system assaults the thyroid gland, causing inflammation and reduced function.

2. **Iodine Deficiency:** Inadequate dietary intake of iodine, a key ingredient for thyroid hormone production, might lead to hypothyroidism.

3. **Thyroid Surgery or Radiation Treatment:** Surgical removal of the thyroid gland or radiation treatment to the neck region might result in hypothyroidism.

4. **Medicines:** Certain medicines, such as lithium, amiodarone, and several anti-thyroid treatments, might interfere with thyroid hormone synthesis.

5. **Pituitary or Hypothalamic Dysfunction:** Disorders affecting the pituitary gland or hypothalamus may disrupt the HPT axis and compromise thyroid function.

Relationship Between Thyroid Health and Perimenopause

The link between thyroid health and perimenopause is nuanced and multifaceted, since both thyroid function and the menopausal transition may impact one other's results and symptoms.

1. **Thyroid Function during Perimenopause:** Hormonal Fluctuations: Perimenopause is marked by variable levels of oestrogen and progesterone. These hormonal changes may impact thyroid hormone production and metabolism. Oestrogen, in particular, has a function in regulating thyroid hormone-binding proteins and the conversion

of thyroxine (T4) to the more active triiodothyronine (T3).

2. **Thyroid Autoimmunity:** Perimenopause may also correlate with an increased risk of thyroid autoimmune illnesses, such as Hashimoto's thyroiditis. Autoimmune thyroiditis may lead to inflammation and damage to the thyroid gland, affecting thyroid hormone production and leading to hypothyroidism.

Impact of Thyroid Dysfunction on Perimenopause

Menstrual Irregularities: Thyroid disorder, especially hypothyroidism, may interrupt the menstrual cycle and lead to irregular periods, severe bleeding, or amenorrhea (lack of menstruation). These monthly changes may increase the issues of perimenopause.

1. **Hormonal Symptoms:** Symptoms of thyroid dysfunction, such as tiredness, weight gain, mood changes, and cognitive impairment, might overlap with those often observed during perimenopause. Women with misdiagnosed or poorly treated thyroid

problems may ascribe their symptoms only to perimenopause, leading to underrecognition and undertreatment of thyroid issues.

2. **Exacerbation of Menopausal Symptoms:** Thyroid disease may increase menopausal symptoms, such as hot flashes, night sweats, sleep disorders, and mood changes. Women with both perimenopause and thyroid issues may suffer more severe or persistent menopausal symptoms compared to those with normal thyroid function.

3. **Cardiovascular Risk:** Hypothyroidism, if left untreated, may raise the risk of cardiovascular disease, including high cholesterol levels, hypertension, and atherosclerosis. Perimenopause alone is related to increases in cardiovascular risk factors, and the presence of thyroid disease may further aggravate these concerns.

Diagnosis and Management

1. **Challenges in Diagnosis:** The overlap in symptoms between perimenopause and thyroid disease might provide complications

in diagnosis. Healthcare practitioners should retain a high index of suspicion for thyroid issues in women presenting with suggestive symptoms during perimenopause and do extensive examinations, including thyroid function testing.

2. **Optimising Thyroid Function:** Effective care of thyroid dysfunction during perimenopause entails optimising thyroid hormone levels with hormone replacement therapy (e.g., levothyroxine for hypothyroidism) and treating underlying autoimmune processes (e.g., Hashimoto's thyroiditis). Individualised treatment approaches should incorporate characteristics such as age, comorbidities, drug interactions, and patient preferences.

3. **Lifestyle Modifications:** Healthy lifestyle behaviours, including a balanced diet, frequent exercise, stress management, and appropriate sleep, may enhance thyroid health and general well-being throughout perimenopause. Avoiding recognised causes of thyroid autoimmunity, such as high iodine

consumption or exposure to environmental pollutants, may also be useful.

Symptoms, Diagnosis, and Treatment Options

Symptoms of Hypothyroidism: Hypothyroidism may appear with a broad variety of symptoms, which may vary in severity and presentation. Common symptoms include:

- Fatigue - Weight gain
- Cold intolerance
- Dry skin and hair
- Constipation
- Muscle weakness
- Joint pain
- Depression
- Memory impairment
- Menstrual irregularity
- Hoarseness
- Slow heart rate
- Elevated cholesterol levels

Diagnosis of Hypothyroidism: Diagnosing hypothyroidism includes a mix of clinical examination, thyroid function testing, and imaging techniques.

Thyroid Function Tests:
- **TSH (Thyroid-Stimulating Hormone):** Elevated TSH values indicate hypothyroidism, whereas lower levels imply hyperthyroidism.
- **Free T4 (Thyroxine):** Low free T4 levels accompany hypothyroidism, while increased levels are found in hyperthyroidism.
- **Thyroid Antibody Tests:** Detect the presence of antibodies linked with autoimmune thyroid illnesses, such as Hashimoto's thyroiditis and Graves' disease.

Treatment Options for Hypothyroidism
- **Levothyroxine Replacement Therapy:** Synthetic T4 hormone replacement therapy is the primary treatment for hypothyroidism. Dosage is titrated depending on TSH levels and individual response.
- **Lifestyle Modifications:** Healthy lifestyle choices, including a balanced diet, frequent exercise, stress management, and appropriate

sleep, may promote thyroid health and enhance treatment effects.

- **Regular Monitoring:** Periodic monitoring of thyroid function tests is required to evaluate treatment response and modify medication dose as needed.

Chapter 5: Nutrition and Supplements

As women navigate the perimenopause era, they frequently confront numerous physical and emotional obstacles, making it vital to prioritise their health via food choices and additional assistance.

Nutrition plays a critical role in promoting general health and well-being during perimenopause, a transitional period distinguished by hormonal swings and physiological changes. Here are numerous reasons why emphasising diet is vital during perimenopause:

1. **Hormonal Balance:** Nutrient-dense meals contain vital vitamins, minerals, and phytonutrients that promote hormonal balance. Adequate consumption of minerals including vitamin B6, magnesium, and omega-3 fatty acids may help balance hormone production and reduce symptoms such as mood swings, hot flashes, and irregular periods.

2. **Bone Health:** Perimenopause is connected with a fall in oestrogen levels, which may raise the risk of osteoporosis and bone fractures. Calcium, vitamin D, vitamin K, and other bone-supporting minerals are crucial for maintaining bone density and minimising the risk of osteoporosis throughout this stage of life.

3. **Heart Health:** As oestrogen levels fall during perimenopause, women may suffer alterations in cholesterol levels and an increased risk of cardiovascular disease. A heart-healthy diet rich in fruits, vegetables, whole grains, lean meats, and healthy fats may help regulate cholesterol levels, blood

pressure, and inflammation, decreasing the risk of heart disease.

4. **Weight Management:** Many women suffer weight gain or changes in body composition during perimenopause, generally owing to hormonal fluctuations, slowed metabolism, and lifestyle factors. A balanced diet that emphasises on nutrient-rich meals and portion control may assist good weight management and metabolism throughout this period.

5. **Energy and vigour:** Nutrient-rich diets give the energy and vigour required to sustain the body's changing demands throughout perimenopause. Consuming a mix of fruits, vegetables, whole grains, lean proteins, and healthy fats may help preserve energy levels, boost mood, and promote overall well-being.

6. **Gut Health:** The gut microbiota has a crucial role in immune function, digestion, and nutritional absorption. Including fibre-rich foods, probiotics, and prebiotics in the diet may improve gut health, decrease bloating,

and relieve digestive symptoms typically reported during perimenopause, such as constipation and bloating.

7. **Mental Health and Cognitive performance:** Nutrition has a tremendous influence on mental health and cognitive performance. Consuming omega-3 fatty acids, antioxidants, and other brain-supporting nutrients may help promote mood control, decrease anxiety and sadness, and boost cognitive performance during perimenopause.

8. **Overall Well-Being:** Optimal diet is critical for sustaining overall health, vitality, and quality of life throughout perimenopause. A well-balanced diet that satisfies dietary demands and supports important physiological systems may help women traverse this transitional time with improved resilience, energy, and vitality.

Dietary Recommendations for Managing Symptoms during Perimenopause

Adopting a well-balanced diet customised to support hormonal balance and general health may greatly ease symptoms and promote well-being.

1. **Increase Intake of Phytoestrogens:** Phytoestrogens are plant-derived chemicals that demonstrate oestrogen-like effects in the body. Including phytoestrogen-rich foods in your diet may help alleviate symptoms linked with decreased oestrogen levels during perimenopause.
   Sources of phytoestrogens include soybeans, tofu, tempeh, edamame, flaxseeds, sesame seeds, lentils, chickpeas, and whole grains like oats and barley.

2. **Emphasise Whole Foods:** Focus on eating a range of whole, unprocessed foods to deliver critical nutrients and antioxidants that promote general health and hormonal balance.

Incorporate lots of fruits, vegetables, whole grains, lean proteins (such as chicken, fish, tofu, beans, and lentils), nuts, seeds, and healthy fats (found in avocados, olive oil, and fatty fish like salmon and mackerel) into your daily meals.

3. **Prioritise Calcium-Rich Foods:** Calcium is crucial for bone health, and women going through perimenopause are at higher risk of bone loss. Ensure appropriate calcium intake by including calcium-rich items in your diet. Good sources of calcium include dairy products (such as milk, yoghurt, and cheese), fortified plant-based milk substitutes, leafy greens (including kale, collard greens, and broccoli), almonds, and tofu.

4. **Optimise Vitamin D Intake:** Vitamin D is vital for calcium absorption and bone health. Adequate vitamin D levels are particularly crucial for women during perimenopause. Get vitamin D via sun exposure (but be cautious of skin protection measures), fortified dairy or plant-based milk, fatty fish

(such as salmon and tuna), egg yolks, and vitamin D supplements if required.

5. **Manage Blood Sugar Levels:** Fluctuations in hormone levels during perimenopause might alter blood sugar management. Focus on having a balanced diet that contains complex carbs, fibre-rich foods, lean proteins, and healthy fats to help stabilise blood sugar levels.

   Choose whole grains (such as quinoa, brown rice, and whole wheat), fruits, vegetables, legumes, nuts, seeds, and lean proteins (such as chicken, turkey, fish, tofu, and beans) as part of your meals.

6. **Stay Hydrated:** Adequate hydration is vital for general health and well-being during perimenopause. Drink lots of water throughout the day to keep hydrated and support body functioning.

   Aim to drink at least 8-10 glasses of water daily, and increase your fluid consumption if you're exercising or in hot weather.

7. **Limit Processed Foods and Added Sugars:** Processed foods, sugary snacks, and refined carbs may worsen hormone imbalances, promote inflammation, and contribute to weight gain and mood swings.

   Minimise intake of sweet treats, processed snacks, white bread, sugary cereals, sugary drinks, and other refined carbs.

8. **Consider Herbal Supplements and Teas:** Certain herbal supplements and teas may give symptom alleviation and enhance general well-being during perimenopause.

   Examples include black cohosh, evening primrose oil, red clover, dong quai, and herbal teas such as chamomile, peppermint, and lemon balm. However, it's vital to talk with a healthcare expert before utilising herbal supplements, particularly if you have current medical issues or are taking drugs.

9. **Moderate Caffeine and Alcohol Intake:** Caffeine and alcohol use might increase symptoms including hot flashes, mood swings, and sleeplessness in certain women. Limit your consumption of caffeinated

beverages and alcoholic drinks, particularly if they increase your symptoms.

Opt for decaffeinated alternatives or herbal teas if you're sensitive to caffeine, and take alcohol in moderation.

10. **Listen to Your Body:** Pay attention to how various meals and drinks impact your symptoms and general well-being. Keep a food journal to document your consumption and symptoms, and alter your diet appropriately.

    Every woman's experience of perimenopause is unique, so it's crucial to listen to your body and make nutritional choices that fit your specific requirements and preferences.

Meal Planning and Healthy Eating Strategies during Perimenopause

Meal planning and implementing healthy eating techniques are crucial components of controlling symptoms and increasing general well-being during perimenopause. By integrating nutrient-rich meals, balancing macronutrients, and exercising mindful eating practices, women may improve their nutritional intake and maintain hormonal balance. Here's a guide on meal planning and healthy eating practices to consider:

1. **Meal Planning Tips:** Set Realistic Goals: Establish reasonable objectives for meal planning, considering your time, culinary abilities, and nutritional preferences. Start with tiny, doable measures and progressively include healthier alternatives in your meals.

2. **Plan Ahead:** Take time to plan your meals for the week, including breakfast, lunch, supper, and snacks. Create a shopping list based on your meal plan to ensure you have all the required products on hand.

3. **Focus on Nutrient-Rich Foods:** Prioritise full, unprocessed foods such as fruits, vegetables, whole grains, lean meats, and healthy fats. Aim to incorporate a diversity of colours and textures in your meals to optimise nutritional uptake.

4. **Balance Macronutrients:** Aim for a balanced distribution of macronutrients in

each meal, including carbs, protein, and healthy fats. Incorporate complex carbs, lean proteins, and fibre-rich meals to enhance energy levels, satiety, and blood sugar regulation.

5. **Practice Portion Control:** Pay attention to portion sizes and avoid excessive meals, which may lead to excess calorie consumption and weight gain. Use smaller plates and utensils to help limit portion sizes and avoid overeating.

6. **Prepare Meals in Advance:** Consider batch cooking or preparing meals in advance to save time on hectic weekdays. Cook huge amounts of soups, stews, or casseroles that can be portioned up and saved for future meals.

7. **Include a Variety of Flavors and Textures:** Experiment with various herbs, spices, and seasonings to improve the flavour of your meals without depending on excessive salt or sugar. Incorporate a range of textures, such as

crisp veggies, soft meats, and chewy grains, to make your meals more pleasurable.

8. **Keep Hydrated:** Drink lots of water throughout the day to keep hydrated and help digestion. Limit intake of sugary beverages and caffeinated drinks, opting for water, herbal teas, or infused water instead.

Healthy Eating Strategies

1. **Mindful Eating:** Practise mindful eating by paying attention to hunger and fullness signals, eating deliberately, and savouring each meal. Avoid distractions like screens or work during meals, enabling yourself to completely participate in the dining experience.

2. **Listen to Your Body:** Tune into your body's cues and change your dietary habits appropriately. Eat when you're hungry and stop when you're full, avoiding mindless snacking or emotional eating.

3. **Eat Regularly:** Aim to eat frequent meals and snacks throughout the day to maintain

stable blood sugar levels and minimise energy dumps. Include a mix of carbs, protein, and healthy fats in each meal to maintain sustained energy and satiety.

4. **Include Protein at Every Meal:** Incorporate protein-rich foods such as lean meats, chicken, fish, tofu, beans, lentils, Greek yoghurt, and eggs into your meals to promote muscular health, metabolism, and hormone balance.

5. **Prioritise Fiber-Rich Foods:** Include enough of fibre-rich foods such as fruits, vegetables, whole grains, legumes, nuts, and seeds in your diet to assist digestion, regulate bowel movements, and encourage feelings of fullness.

6. **Limit Processed Foods and Added Sugars:** Minimise intake of processed foods, sugary snacks, and refined carbs, which may disrupt hormone balance, raise inflammation, and lead to weight gain and mood swings.

7. **Practice Portion Control:** Be conscious of portion sizes and avoid excessive quantities, particularly of calorie-dense items like sweets, fried foods, and high-fat snacks. Use smaller plates and utensils to help limit portion sizes and avoid overeating.

Tested and Proven: Seven-Day Meal Plan to Get You Started

Day 1:

Breakfast: Greek yoghourt with berries and almonds

Snack: Carrot sticks with hummus

Lunch: Quinoa salad with mixed vegetables and grilled chicken

Snack: Apple slices with peanut butter

Dinner: Baked salmon with roasted sweet potatoes and steamed broccoli

Day 2:

Breakfast: Spinach and feta omelette with whole grain toast

Snack: Greek yoghourt with sliced banana and honey
Lunch: Lentil soup with whole grain crackers
Snack: Trail mix (nuts, seeds, dried fruits)
Dinner: Stir-fried tofu with mixed vegetables and brown rice

Day 3:

Breakfast: Overnight oats with chia seeds, almond milk, and sliced strawberries
Snack: Cottage cheese with pineapple chunks
Lunch: Turkey and avocado wrap with mixed greens
Snack: Celery sticks with almond butter
Dinner: Grilled shrimp skewers with quinoa pilaf and roasted vegetables

Day 4:

Breakfast: Whole grain cereal with almond milk and sliced peaches
Snack: Edamame with sea salt
Lunch: Chickpea salad with cucumbers, tomatoes, and feta cheese
Snack: Bell pepper strips with guacamole

Dinner: Baked chicken breast with mashed sweet potatoes and sautéed spinach

Day 5:

Breakfast: Banana smoothie with spinach, almond milk, and protein powder
Snack: Hard-boiled egg with cherry tomatoes
Lunch: Vegetable stir-fry with tofu and brown rice
Snack: Greek yoghourts with granola
Dinner: Turkey chilli with mixed beans and side salad

Day 6:

Breakfast: Whole grain toast with avocado and poached eggs
Snack: Cottage cheese with mixed berries
Lunch: Quinoa and black bean salad with avocado dressing
Snack: Almonds and dried apricots
Dinner: Baked cod with roasted vegetables and quinoa

Day 7:

Breakfast: Oatmeal with sliced apples, cinnamon, and walnuts

Snack: Hummus with cucumber slices

Lunch: Spinach salad with grilled chicken, strawberries, and balsamic vinaigrette

Snack: Greek yoghourt with honey and almonds

Dinner: Lentil curry with brown rice and steamed broccoli

Chapter 6: Alcohol, Caffeine, and Perimenopause

Alcohol and caffeine are regularly used substances that may have considerable impacts on hormonal balance, especially during the perimenopausal period. Understanding their effect on oestrogen and progesterone levels and their effect on perimenopausal symptoms is vital for women navigating this transitional phase.

Effects on Oestrogen and Progesterone Levels

Alcohol:
1. Alcohol drinking may affect oestrogen levels in women. Chronic alcohol drinking may lead

to an increase in oestrogen production since alcohol interferes with the liver's capacity to metabolise oestrogen properly.

2. Conversely, high alcohol intake may also suppress oestrogen levels by decreasing ovarian function and blocking the production of gonadotropins, hormones that stimulate the ovaries to generate oestrogen.

3. Additionally, alcohol may alter the equilibrium between oestrogen and progesterone by interfering with the synthesis and metabolism of progesterone, resulting in hormonal abnormalities.

Caffeine:

1. Caffeine use has been connected with variations in oestrogen and progesterone levels, but the processes are not completely understood.

2. Some studies show that coffee may boost oestrogen levels by stimulating the adrenal glands to create more cortisol, a stress

hormone that may indirectly alter oestrogen production.

3. On the other side, caffeine has also been discovered to limit the absorption of magnesium, a mineral that plays a role in oestrogen metabolism, perhaps leading to reduced oestrogen levels.

Influence on Perimenopausal Symptoms

Alcohol:

Alcohol intake has been related to an increased risk of various perimenopausal symptoms, including:

1. **Hot flashes:** Alcohol may widen blood vessels and raise body temperature, worsening hot flashes and nocturnal sweats.
2. **Mood Swings and Depression:** Alcohol is a central nervous system depressant that may increase mood disturbances and depressive symptoms in vulnerable persons.
3. **Sleep difficulties:** While alcohol may initially induce relaxation and tiredness, it may alter sleep patterns and lead to

fragmented sleep, increasing insomnia and sleep disorders typical during perimenopause.

4. **Weight Gain:** Alcohol is rich in calories and may lead to weight gain, which may aggravate symptoms such as bloating and exhaustion.

Caffeine:

Caffeine use may also affect perimenopausal symptoms in numerous ways:

1. **Night sweats and hot flashes:** Caffeine has thermogenic effects that might elevate body temperature and provoke hot flashes and night sweats in certain women.
2. **Mood disturbances:** Excessive coffee consumption may worsen anxiety, irritability, and mood swings, which are frequent perimenopausal symptoms.
3. **Insomnia and sleep disturbances:** Caffeine is a stimulant that may interfere with sleep onset and quality, leading to insomnia and interrupted sleep patterns.
4. **Bone health:** High caffeine consumption has been related to reduced calcium absorption and increased urine calcium excretion, which may adversely affect bone density and raise

the   risk   of   osteoporosis   during perimenopause.

Strategies for Moderating Alcohol and Caffeine Consumption during Perimenopause

Moderating alcohol and caffeine use is vital for women navigating perimenopause to promote hormonal balance and reduce the worsening of symptoms. Implementing techniques to restrict intake may assist women in maintaining their general health and well-being throughout this time. Here are some successful ways to reduce alcohol and caffeine consumption:

1. **Set Explicit Limits:** Establish explicit rules for alcohol and caffeine intake based on prescribed limits and personal preferences. Define the exact amounts and frequency of intake that fit with your health objectives and perimenopausal symptoms.

2. **Monitor Intake:** Keep track of your alcohol and caffeine usage by documenting the quantity and frequency of drinks consumed

each day. Use a notebook or smartphone app to track your intake and uncover trends or triggers that may lead to excessive eating.

3. **Practise Conscious Drinking:** Be conscious of your motives for drinking alcohol and caffeine and the possible influence on your health and well-being. Pause and examine your desires or impulses before reaching for a drink, and seek healthier options or coping skills to address underlying needs or emotions.

4. **Choose Quality over Quantity:** Opt for high-quality alcoholic drinks and caffeine sources that deliver more pleasure and enjoyment with fewer amounts. Select quality wines, craft beers, or specialty coffees that you can relish and appreciate without having to drink enormous amounts.

5. **Set limits:** Establish limits around alcohol and caffeine usage to prevent peer pressure or social factors that may lead to overindulgence. Communicate your limitations and preferences to friends, family,

and social circles, and seek out supportive situations that respect your choices.

6. **Plan:** Plan for social gatherings or activities where alcohol and caffeine may be present by outlining objectives and techniques for moderation. Bring your non-alcoholic drinks or herbal teas to enjoy as alternatives, and be prepared to respectfully refuse offers of alcohol or caffeine if they exceed your limitations.

7. **Alternate with Water:** Alternate alcoholic and caffeinated drinks with water or other non-alcoholic, hydrating choices to moderate your consumption and lessen total intake. Sipping water between drinks may help attenuate alcohol and caffeine effects and avoid dehydration.

8. **Practice Self-Care:** Prioritise self-care activities such as regular exercise, stress management, appropriate sleep, and good nutrition to enhance general well-being and lessen dependency on alcohol and caffeine as

coping methods for perimenopausal symptoms.

9. **Seek Support:** Reach out to friends, family, or support groups for encouragement and accountability in decreasing alcohol and caffeine usage. Share your objectives and problems with trustworthy folks who can give help, understanding, and inspiration throughout your path.

10. **Know When to Seek Help:** Be aware of signals of problematic alcohol or caffeine intake, such as dependency, withdrawal symptoms, or harmful effects on physical or mental health. If you struggle to limit intake on your own, get professional support from a healthcare practitioner, therapist, or addiction expert.

Alcohol-Free Alternatives

For women who are trying to decrease their alcohol intake or abstain completely, there are lots of tasty and refreshing alcohol-free options available. These alternatives give the ability to socialise, relax, and enjoy delectable drinks without the possible detrimental effects of alcohol on hormonal balance and general health. Here are some alcohol-free options that are excellent for perimenopausal women:

1. **Mocktails:** Mocktails are non-alcoholic beverages that replicate the tastes and appearance of classic cocktails without the alcohol content. They may be produced with several components, including fresh fruits, herbs, juices, sparkling water, and flavoured syrups. Popular mocktails include virgin mojitos, pina coladas, margaritas, and spritzers.

2. **Herbal Teas:** Herbal teas are caffeine-free drinks prepared from dried herbs, flowers, fruits, and spices steeped in hot water. They come in a broad variety of tastes and variations, such as chamomile, peppermint, ginger, hibiscus, and rooibos. Herbal teas are not only calming and hydrating but also provide possible health advantages, including stress reduction and digestive assistance.

3. **Sparkling Water:** Sparkling water, often known as soda water or seltzer, is carbonated water laced with bubbles for a delightful and bubbly feel. It may be eaten simply or flavoured with natural extracts, fruit essences, or herbal infusions. Sparkling water is a hydrating and calorie-free alternative to sugary sodas and alcoholic drinks, making it a perfect option for perimenopausal women.

4. **Fruit Infusions:** Fruit infusions entail infusing water with fresh fruits, vegetables, herbs, and spices to give a natural taste and fragrance without added sugars or artificial substances. Simply add sliced fruits like berries, citrus, melons, or cucumbers to a pitcher of water and let it soak for a few hours in the refrigerator. The outcome is a delightful and hydrating beverage filled with taste and nutrition.

5. **Kombucha:** Kombucha is a fermented tea beverage prepared from sweetened tea that has been fermented with a symbiotic culture of bacteria and yeast (SCOBY). It has a somewhat acidic and effervescent tasting

profile and is available in a range of flavours, such as ginger, berry, and citrus. Kombucha is rich in bacteria and antioxidants, delivering possible digestive and immunological support advantages.

6. **Virgin Mary:** A Virgin Mary is a non-alcoholic variant of the popular Bloody Mary drink, prepared with tomato juice, lemon or lime juice, Worcestershire sauce, spicy sauce, and different ingredients. It may be modified to suit different preferences by altering the spice level and adding garnishes like celery sticks, olives, pickles, or bacon.

7. **Iced Herbal Lemonades:** Iced herbal lemonades blend freshly squeezed lemon juice with herbal infusions, sweeteners, and ice for a pleasant and nourishing beverage. Experiment with various herbal combinations such as lavender, mint, basil, or rosemary to produce distinct flavour profiles that tantalise the taste receptors.

8. **Coconut Water:** Coconut water is the clear liquid found within young green coconuts

and is naturally rich in electrolytes, vitamins, and minerals. It has a somewhat sweet and nutty taste and may be consumed chilled or blended with other fruit juices for extra flavour. Coconut water is hydrating and nourishing, making it a perfect option for post-exercise recovery or hot weather hydration.

Responsible Drinking During Perimenopause: What to do

Responsible drinking entails conscious intake of alcohol to limit the possible negative consequences on hormonal balance, symptom severity, and general health. While moderate alcohol consumption may be okay for some women, it's crucial to approach drinking with awareness, moderation, and consideration of individual requirements and sensitivities. Here are some recommendations for careful drinking during perimenopause:

1. **Know Your limitations:** Understand your body's tolerance for alcohol and know your limitations. Recognize how much alcohol you can safely drink without suffering bad

consequences on your physical or emotional well-being.

2. **Set Clear limits:** Establish clear limits surrounding alcohol use based on personal preferences, health objectives, and perimenopausal symptoms. Decide on particular boundaries for the number, frequency, and sort of alcoholic drinks you're comfortable ingesting.

3. **Pace Yourself:** Pace your alcohol intake by drinking drinks slowly and alternating with non-alcoholic liquids like water or herbal tea. Avoid drinking too rapidly or engaging in drinking activities that promote rapid intake.

4. **Choose Quality over Quantity:** Opt for high-quality alcoholic drinks created with premium ingredients and skill. Select smaller portions of top-shelf liquors, craft beers, or boutique wines that give more pleasure and satisfaction with less volume.

5. **Be Attentive to Some Factors:** Be attentive to emotional, social, or environmental factors

that may impact your drinking habit. Identify events, emotions, or societal pressures that entice you to drink excessively and learn coping methods to handle these triggers successfully.

6. **Practice Moderation:** Practice moderation by restricting your alcohol consumption to a reasonable quantity on every occasion. Follow suggested standards for moderate drinking, which normally include up to one standard drink per day for women.

7. **Listen to Your Body:** Listen to your body's signals and pay attention to how alcohol impacts your physical and mental well-being. Notice any changes in mood, energy levels, sleep quality, digestion, or perimenopausal symptoms after consuming alcohol.

8. **Prioritise Hydration:** Stay hydrated by drinking lots of water before, during, and after ingesting alcohol. Alcohol is dehydrating and may increase symptoms like hot flashes, headaches, and weariness, so it's crucial to refill fluids periodically.

9. **Plan Ahead:** Plan for social gatherings or occasions where alcohol will be present by outlining objectives and methods for safe drinking. Decide in advance how many drinks you'll have and stick to your plan to prevent overindulging.

10. **Know When to Stop:** Know when to stop drinking and identify the indications of drunkenness, such as impaired judgement, slurred speech, unsteady walking, or lack of coordination. Stop drinking if you feel inebriated or if you've surpassed your planned limit.

11. **Monitor Your Health:** Monitor your physical and mental health periodically and be alert of any changes or symptoms that may occur from alcohol usage. Consult with a healthcare practitioner if you have concerns about your drinking habits or if you suffer unfavourable impacts on your health or well-being.

12. **Eat Before Consuming:** Consume a balanced meal before consuming alcohol to assist slow down the absorption of alcohol into your system. Eating meals may also help lower the likelihood of having unpleasant symptoms such as nausea, dizziness, or hypoglycemia.

13. **Avoid Mixing Alcohol with Medicines:** Avoid mixing alcohol with medicines, including over-the-counter and prescription pharmaceuticals, since it may interfere with their efficacy and lead to harmful interactions. Consult with your healthcare practitioner or pharmacist to learn whether it's okay to consume alcohol while taking drugs.

14. **Be Aware of Hormonal Sensitivity:** Be aware that hormonal variations during perimenopause may enhance sensitivity to alcohol and its consequences. Women may discover that they have a lesser tolerance for alcohol at this period, so it's vital to drink thoughtfully and adjust intake accordingly.

15. **Use Alcohol-Free Days:** Incorporate alcohol-free days into your week to give your body a vacation from drinking and encourage balance and moderation. Aim for at least two to three alcohol-free days each week to improve general health and well-being.

16. **Educate Yourself About Alcohol Units:** Educate yourself about standard alcohol units and how they relate to various kinds and volumes of alcoholic drinks. Understanding alcohol units might help you manage your consumption more efficiently and make educated choices about drinking.

Chapter 7: Sex and Intimacy During Perimenopause

Most women know that menopause comes with a few obstacles when it comes to sexual health, but what a lot of women don't realise is that those concerns may begin during perimenopause – the months and years before menopause begins. Even for women who believe they're prepared for "the change of life," changes in their sexual desire and sexual comfort might be unexpected and even a bit discouraging.

Fortunately, you may do numerous things to reclaim sexual pleasure throughout the years leading up to menopause (and during menopause, too).

This phase may bring about variations in libido, vaginal health, and emotional well-being, altering sexual desire, pleasure, and closeness with partners. Understanding the complexity of sex and intimacy during perimenopause is vital for women and their partners to manage this era with openness, communication, and resilience.

During perimenopause, many women experience changes in their sexual wants and reactions owing to hormone variations, changes in body image, and other physical and mental variables. While some women may experience a drop in libido or changes in arousal patterns, others may find that their sexual urges stay constant or even grow. Additionally, perimenopause may bring about changes in vaginal health, such as dryness, irritation, and pain during intercourse, which can further influence sexual pleasure and closeness.

Despite these limitations, perimenopause also brings chances for development, discovery, and greater connection in sexual interactions. By adopting open communication, mutual understanding, and a willingness to adjust to shifting wants and desires, couples may manage perimenopause with grace and compassion, creating intimacy and connection in new and meaningful ways.

Strategies for Managing Changes in Libido and Sexual Function

1. **Hormone Replacement Therapy (HRT):** Consider hormone replacement treatment (HRT) under the advice of a healthcare expert to reduce symptoms of vaginal dryness, pain, and decreased libido. HRT may help restore hormonal balance and enhance sexual performance in some women suffering perimenopausal symptoms.

2. **Vaginal Moisturisers and Lubricants:** Use over-the-counter vaginal moisturisers and lubricants to reduce vaginal dryness and pain during intercourse. These items may give brief relief and increase sexual enjoyment by improving lubrication and minimising friction.

3. **Pelvic Floor Exercises:** Practise pelvic floor exercises, commonly known as Kegel exercises, to strengthen pelvic muscles and

increase vaginal tone and sensitivity. Pelvic floor exercises may help decrease symptoms of urine incontinence, improve sexual function, and boost orgasmic response during perimenopause.

4. **Healthy Lifestyle Habits:** Adopt a healthy lifestyle that includes regular exercise, balanced eating, stress management, and appropriate sleep to promote hormone balance and general well-being. Maintaining a healthy weight, avoiding smoking, and limiting alcohol use might help enhance sexual function and desire during perimenopause.

5. **Sexual Counseling or Therapy:** Seek treatment from a trained sex therapist or counsellor to address psychological and emotional reasons leading to changes in desire and sexual function. Sexual counselling or therapy may give a safe environment to examine problems, better communication with partners, and build coping mechanisms for managing sexual difficulties during perimenopause.

6. **Exploring Alternative Closeness:** Explore non-penetrative sexual practices, such as sensual massage, reciprocal masturbation, or oral sex, to preserve closeness and enjoyment with partners. Experimenting with new sexual methods, positions, or fantasies may help revive desire and excitement in the bedroom during perimenopause.

7. **Experimenting with Sensual Aids:** Consider using sensual aids such as sex toys, sexy books, or erotic movies to boost arousal and enjoyment during sexual activity. Sensual aids may give extra stimulation and diversity, boosting sexual pleasure and enjoyment for women and their partners.

8. **Medication Review:** Review medicines with a healthcare professional to identify any drugs that may be related to sexual dysfunction or low libido. Some drugs, such as antidepressants, antihistamines, and blood pressure medications, might impact sexual performance and may need changes or alternate choices.

9. **Mindfulness and Relaxation Techniques:** Practise mindfulness and relaxation methods such as deep breathing, meditation, or yoga to decrease tension and increase relaxation. Stress reduction may help ease anxiety and tension, improve mood, and boost sexual desire and responsiveness.

10. **Discussion with Spouse:** Engage in open and honest discussion with your spouse regarding changes in libido and sexual function during perimenopause. Share your thoughts, worries, and wishes freely, and urge your spouse to do the same. Mutual understanding, empathy, and support may increase the emotional connection and closeness in your relationship.

11. **Sensate Focus Exercises:** Try sensate focus exercises as a means to strengthen intimacy and connection with your mate. These exercises entail non-sexual contact and exploration of each other's bodies, concentrating on feelings and enjoyment rather than performance or climax. Sensate

attention may help create trust, closeness, and excitement, creating the framework for enjoyable sexual encounters.

12. **Explore Erotica and Fantasy:** Explore erotica, books, or films that engage your imagination and kindle desire. Engaging in erotic fantasies or role-playing with your spouse may boost sexual desire and pleasure, providing freshness and variation to your personal experiences.

13. **Practice Patience and Self-Compassion:** Practise patience and self-compassion as you negotiate changes in libido and sexual function throughout perimenopause. Understand that it's natural to have swings in sexual desire and responsiveness during this transitional time and be kind to yourself while you explore ways to handle these changes.

14. **Focus on closeness Beyond Intercourse:** Focus on closeness and connection with your spouse beyond intercourse. Explore alternate types of physical love, such as cuddling,

kissing, or holding hands, to preserve closeness and emotional connection during times when sexual desire may be reduced.

Hormonal Variables that Impact Sexual Function

The menopausal transition is defined by variable oestrogen levels, irregular menstrual cycles, and typically a random blend of oestrogen excess and oestrogen shortage symptoms. Therefore one week a woman can be feeling mastalgia and heavy bleeding and the next, experiencing vasomotor symptoms, sleep problems, and anxiety as a result of oestrogen shortage. These hormonal changes will have a major influence on the woman's sexual desire and ability to get aroused and/or attain orgasm.

Vaginal atrophy is a result of postmenopausal oestrogen insufficiency, however since oestrogen levels are normally maintained until the last menstrual month, most perimenopausal women remain unaffected. During the perimenopause, women commonly complain of vaginal dryness in connection to sexual activity. Rather than being owing to oestrogen inadequacy, this is an indication of an inability to get aroused and lubricated. In this circumstance, therapy with vaginal oestrogen does not address the condition.

In contrast to the reduction in oestrogen after menopause, testosterone levels do not alter suddenly over the menopause transition but diminish slowly with age from the mid-reproductive years. Studies of testosterone treatment have not been undertaken in perimenopausal women. However, therapy of women in their late reproductive years and postmenopausal women with testosterone has been related to greater arousal and vaginal lubrication and decreased dyspareunia. Testosterone levels originate from ovarian testosterone synthesis and conversion of adrenal dehydroepiandrosterone SDHEAT to testosterone in the target tissues.

Maintaining Intimacy and Connection

Emotional closeness and sexual connection are what nurture a relationship and maintain the shine of sensuality and desire.

Perimenopause may bring barriers to intimacy and connection in partnerships. However, with open conversation, sensitivity, and a willingness to adjust, couples may manage this transitional phase and improve their partnership. Let's examine ways to keep closeness and connection throughout perimenopause:

1. **Open Communication:** Open and honest communication is the cornerstone of intimacy and connection in any relationship, particularly during perimenopause. Encourage discussion with your spouse about your emotions, worries, and needs relating to intimacy and sexual health. Share your experiences with perimenopausal symptoms, such as changes in libido, vaginal dryness, or mood swings, and allow your spouse to share their views and emotions as well. Establishing a safe and supportive environment for conversation helps build understanding, empathy, and mutual support in experiencing perimenopause together.

2. **Empathy and Understanding:** Perimenopause affects both parties in a relationship but in different ways. Practice empathy and compassion towards one other's experiences and struggles throughout this transitional era. Recognize that hormonal

variations, physical changes, and emotional upheavals may affect your partner's libido, mood, and general well-being. Show compassion and support by listening intently, acknowledging their emotions, and providing comfort. By recognising and accepting each other's feelings, you may enhance your emotional connection and build a sense of solidarity in confronting perimenopause together.

3. **Mutual Respect and Acceptance:** Embrace each other's originality and distinctiveness, including the changes that occur with perimenopause. Celebrate your partner's qualities, perseverance, and attractiveness, regardless of any physical or hormonal changes they may encounter. Foster mutual respect and acceptance by recognising each other's value, autonomy, and agency in managing perimenopause and its problems. By emphasising respect and acceptance in your relationship, you can create a supportive and powerful atmosphere for intimacy and connection to grow.

4. **Prioritise Emotional Connection:** Intimacy extends beyond physical intimacy and incorporates emotional connection, trust, and vulnerability. Prioritise emotional connection by spending quality time together, participating in meaningful discussions, and exchanging experiences, ambitions, and goals. Show affection via acts of love, generosity, and gratitude, such as hugs, kisses, or meaningful comments. Cultivate a profound feeling of connection by being present, sensitive, and supportive of each other's emotional needs and wants.

5. **Explore Non-Sexual Intimacy:** Intimacy is multidimensional and may be exhibited in different ways beyond sexual engagement. Explore non-sexual forms of closeness, such as hugging, holding hands, or exchanging expressive gestures, to build your emotional ties and connection. Engage in activities that build connection and intimacy, such as cooking together, going on walks, or practising mindfulness or relaxation methods as a pair. By emphasising non-sexual intimacy, you may improve your emotional

connection and boost closeness in your relationship throughout perimenopause.

6. **Adapt and Explore New forms of Intimacy:** Be open to adjusting and exploring new forms of intimacy that accommodate changes in libido, sexual function, and physical comfort during perimenopause. Experiment with varied types of sexual expressions, such as sensual massage, reciprocal masturbation, or erotic dreams, that prioritise pleasure, connection, and mutual fulfilment. Focus on mutual enjoyment and discovery rather than performance or obtaining certain objectives. By embracing flexibility and inventiveness in your encounters, you may maintain a healthy and gratifying sex life throughout perimenopause.

7. **Seek Professional treatment if Needed:** If issues in sustaining intimacy and connection remain despite your efforts, consider obtaining professional treatment from a therapist, counsellor, or sex therapist. These specialists may give help, skills, and methods

for managing marital challenges, boosting communication, and overcoming sexual concerns during perimenopause. Therapy or counselling may give a safe and supportive environment to examine your thoughts, wants, and problems as individuals and as a couple, enabling development, healing, and intimacy in your relationship.

Pelvic Floor Health and Exercises

Pelvic floor health is a critical element of general well-being for women, especially during perimenopause. The pelvic floor muscles serve a key role in supporting pelvic organs, managing bladder and bowel function, and contributing to sexual function and enjoyment.

As women move through perimenopause, hormonal changes, childbearing, age, and other factors may impair pelvic floor health, leading to symptoms such as urine incontinence, pelvic organ prolapse, and sexual dysfunction. Incorporating pelvic floor exercises into a regular programme may help strengthen these muscles, enhance pelvic floor function, and decrease symptoms associated with pelvic floor dysfunction. Let's go into the intricacies of pelvic floor health and workouts during perimenopause:

1. **Understanding the Pelvic Floor:** The pelvic floor is a combination of muscles, ligaments, and connective tissues that create a supporting hammock-like structure at the bottom of the pelvis. These muscles provide support for pelvic organs, including the bladder, uterus, and rectum, and play a critical role in managing urine and bowel function, as well as sexual function. During perimenopause, hormonal changes and other factors may weaken the pelvic floor muscles, leading to symptoms such as urine incontinence, pelvic organ prolapse, and sexual dysfunction.

2. **Impact of Perimenopause on Pelvic Floor Health:** Hormonal changes during perimenopause, such as decreased oestrogen levels, might impair pelvic floor health by weakening pelvic muscles and connective tissues. Additionally, additional factors such as delivery, obesity, chronic constipation, and

heavy lifting may further strain the pelvic floor muscles, resulting in pelvic floor dysfunction. Common symptoms of pelvic floor dysfunction during perimenopause may include urine incontinence (stress, urge, or mixed), pelvic organ prolapse (bladder, uterus, or rectum sinking into the vaginal canal), pelvic discomfort, and sexual dysfunction.

3. **Importance of Pelvic Floor Exercises:** Pelvic floor exercises, commonly known as Kegel exercises, are aimed to strengthen the pelvic floor muscles, enhance pelvic floor function, and relieve symptoms associated with pelvic floor dysfunction. These exercises include contracting and releasing the pelvic floor muscles to enhance their strength, endurance, and coordination. Regular practice of pelvic floor exercises may help minimise urine incontinence, support pelvic organs, boost sexual function, and improve the general quality of life during perimenopause.

4. **How to Perform Pelvic Floor Exercises:** To conduct pelvic floor exercises:
   - Identify the pelvic floor muscles by thinking that you are attempting to halt the flow of pee or avoid passing gas.
   - Contract the pelvic floor muscles by squeezing and raising them inward and upward.
   - Hold the contraction for a few seconds (target for 5-10 seconds initially) while continuing to breathe normally.
   - Relax the pelvic floor muscles and release the contraction.
   - Repeat the exercise 10-15 times, progressively increasing the length and amount of repetitions as your pelvic floor muscles grow stronger.

5. **Incorporating Pelvic Floor Exercises into Daily Routine:** Pelvic floor exercises may be done discreetly at any time and in any posture, making them simple to include in a daily routine. You may practise pelvic floor exercises while sitting, standing, or lying down, and no additional equipment is necessary.

Try to strive for at least three sets of pelvic floor exercises each day, progressively increasing the time and intensity of each contraction as your pelvic floor muscles develop.

6. **Additional Tips for Pelvic Floor Health:** In addition to pelvic floor exercises, there are numerous more measures you may use to maintain pelvic floor health during perimenopause:

   - Maintain a healthy weight to prevent strain on the pelvic floor muscles.
   - Practise excellent posture and body mechanics to prevent tension on the pelvic floor.
   - Avoid heavy lifting and high-impact activities that may cause pelvic floor dysfunction.
   - Stay hydrated and maintain regular bowel habits to avoid constipation, which may strain the pelvic floor.
   - Seek help from a pelvic health physiotherapist or healthcare practitioner for tailored examination

and treatment of pelvic floor dysfunction.

7. **Advantages of Pelvic Floor Exercises:** Regular practice of pelvic floor exercises provides various advantages for women throughout perimenopause, including:
    - Improved bladder control and less urine incontinence.
    - Prevention or treatment of pelvic organ prolapse.
    - Enhanced sexual function and enjoyment.
    - Alleviation of pelvic pain and discomfort.
    - Increased confidence and quality of life.

Chapter 8: Skin and Hair Care

As women travel through the transforming time of perimenopause, hormonal variations bring about a plethora of changes in their bodies, not just inwardly but also visibly, impacting their skin and hair. The hormonal adjustments observed during perimenopause may contribute to modifications in skin texture, elasticity, and moisture levels, as well as changes in hair growth, thickness, and quality.

These changes may create new problems and necessitate adaptations to skincare and haircare regimens to maintain healthy, bright skin and glossy hair throughout this transitional era of life. In this chapter, we will examine the impact of perimenopause on skin and hair health, address common concerns and issues, and present practical suggestions and methods for improving skincare and haircare routines to boost general well-being and confidence throughout perimenopause.

Common Skin Changes During Perimenopause

Skin changes over a person's lifespan, for both men and women. For women, however, their reproductive hormones substantially impact the skin. Perimenopause is frequently when these skin changes develop, since the fast variations in hormones may result in numerous skin disorders. This leaves many women asking how they might handle menopause and skin changes linked with it. Let's review in depth the most frequent skin changes seen throughout this phase:

1. **Dryness and Dehydration:** One of the most typical skin changes during perimenopause is increased dryness and dehydration. Declining oestrogen levels may lead to reduced oil production in the skin, resulting in dry, flaky, and rough skin texture. Additionally, hormonal imbalances may decrease the skin's capacity to retain moisture, resulting in

greater vulnerability to dryness and moisture loss.

2. **Wrinkles and Fine Lines:** As oestrogen levels diminish during perimenopause, collagen and elastin synthesis in the skin also decrease. Collagen and elastin are important proteins responsible for maintaining skin firmness, elasticity, and smoothness. The decline in these proteins may contribute to the creation of wrinkles, fine lines, and drooping skin, notably around the eyes, lips, and forehead.

3. **Thinning Skin:** Oestrogen plays a critical function in enhancing skin thickness and density by boosting collagen formation and supporting skin cell turnover. As oestrogen levels fall during perimenopause, the skin may become thinner and more delicate, leaving it more prone to bruising, ripping, and damage. Thinning skin may further aggravate the appearance of wrinkles and fine lines.

4. **Age Spots and Hyperpigmentation:** Hormonal variations during perimenopause might lead to the development of age spots, also known as liver spots or sunspots, and hyperpigmentation. Oestrogen has a function in controlling melanin synthesis, the pigment responsible for skin colour. Hormonal imbalances may lead to uneven distribution of melanin in the skin, resulting in the creation of dark spots, patches, or discoloration, especially on sun-exposed regions such as the face, hands, and décolletage.

5. **Acne and Breakouts:** Hormonal variations, especially fluctuations in testosterone levels, might lead to an increase in acne and breakouts during perimenopause. Testosterone promotes sebum production in the skin's oil glands, resulting in increased oil production and clogged pores. Hormonal imbalances may increase acne flare-ups, especially in women who are prone to hormonal acne.

6. **Sensitivity and Irritation:** Changes in hormone levels may also make the skin more sensitive and prone to irritation during perimenopause. Oestrogen helps maintain the skin's protective barrier function, which defends it from environmental aggressors and irritants. Declining oestrogen levels may affect the skin's barrier function, resulting in increased sensitivity, redness, and irritation.

7. **Loss of Elasticity:** Oestrogen is vital for preserving skin elasticity and suppleness by increasing collagen production and blocking collagen breakdown. As oestrogen levels fall during perimenopause, the skin may lose its elasticity and resilience, leading to a loss of firmness and definition. Reduced elasticity may lead to the development of drooping skin and loss of face shape.

8. **Hair Changes:** Hormonal variations during perimenopause may significantly affect hair health and appearance. Some women may have thinning hair, hair loss, or changes in hair structure and quality. Hormonal imbalances, dietary inadequacies, and

hereditary factors may all contribute to hair changes during perimenopause.

Strategies for Maintaining Healthy Skin Care

Maintaining good skin during perimenopause demands a proactive strategy that tackles the particular difficulties given by hormone changes and ageing. By following a thorough skincare regimen suited to the unique requirements of perimenopausal skin, women may successfully treat common skin issues and maintain overall skin health. Here are some recommendations for proper skin care during perimenopause:

1. **Hydration and Moisturization:** Combat dryness and dehydration by including hydrating and moisturising products into your skincare regimen. Choose moderate, non-comedogenic moisturisers designed with components like hyaluronic acid, glycerin, and ceramides to replace moisture levels and improve the skin's natural barrier.

2. **Sun Protection:** Protect your skin from the damaging effects of UV radiation by applying broad-spectrum sunscreen with a least SPF of 30 every day, even on overcast days. Sunscreen helps prevent premature ageing, sunspots, and skin cancer, all of which may be aggravated by hormonal changes during perimenopause.

3. **Gentle Cleansing:** Use a light, non-irritating cleanser to wash your skin twice daily, morning and night. Avoid strong, abrasive cleansers that strip the skin of its natural oils, since they may cause dryness and irritation. Opt for mild, moisturising cleansers that efficiently eliminate pollutants without affecting the skin's moisture barrier.

4. **Anti-Aging Substances:** Incorporate anti-aging substances into your skincare regimen to target fine lines, wrinkles, and loss of elasticity. Look for products containing retinoids, peptides, antioxidants (such as vitamins C and E), and growth factors, which may help increase collagen

synthesis, enhance skin texture, and protect against free radical damage.

5. **Exfoliation:** Exfoliate your skin frequently to eliminate dead skin cells and encourage cell turnover, exposing smoother, more vibrant skin below. Choose mild exfoliants such as alpha hydroxy acids (AHAs) or beta hydroxy acids (BHAs), which may help enhance skin tone and texture without causing irritation or inflammation.

6. **Hormone Replacement Therapy (HRT):** Discuss hormone replacement therapy (HRT) with your healthcare practitioner as a viable option for addressing hormonal imbalances and accompanying skin changes during perimenopause. HRT may help refill diminishing oestrogen levels, increasing skin suppleness, moisture retention, and general skin health.

7. **Nutrient-Rich Diet:** Support skin health from the inside by eating a balanced diet rich in vitamins, minerals, antioxidants, and vital fatty acids. Incorporate foods such as fruits,

vegetables, whole grains, lean proteins, and healthy fats into your diet to supply your skin with the nutrients it needs to maintain maximum health and vitality.

8. **Stress Management:** Practice stress management strategies such as meditation, deep breathing, yoga, or mindfulness to lower stress levels, which may worsen skin concerns and hasten ageing. Chronic stress may stimulate inflammatory reactions in the skin, leading to acne, sensitivity, and other skin issues.

9. **Adequate Sleep:** Prioritise excellent sleep to help your skin to heal and rejuvenate overnight. Aim for 7-8 hours of unbroken sleep each night to maintain healthy skin cell turnover and enhance skin regeneration processes. Lack of sleep may lead to dullness, puffiness, and accelerated ageing of the skin.

10. **Professional Treatments:** Consider professional skincare treatments such as facials, chemical peels, microdermabrasion, or laser therapy to address particular skin

conditions and revitalise the skin. Consult with a dermatologist or skin care professional to identify the most suitable treatments for your skin type and issues.

Hair Loss and Thinning

Hair loss and thinning are typical concerns for women throughout perimenopause, sometimes creating worry and compromising self-esteem. A better understanding of the underlying reasons for these changes and adopting effective treatments is vital for controlling hair health and fostering confidence.

Causes of Hair Loss and Thinning

1. **Genetic Predisposition:** Genetic factors play a crucial role in hair loss and thinning, with certain women being more susceptible to disorders such as female pattern hair loss (androgenetic alopecia). If there is a family history of hair loss or thinning, women may be more prone to encounter similar concerns during perimenopause.

2. **Stress and Anxiety:** Chronic stress and anxiety may promote hair shedding and contribute to hair loss during perimenopause. Stress chemicals such as cortisol may alter the hair development cycle and contribute to telogen effluvium, a disorder marked by excessive loss of hair.

3. **Nutritional Deficiencies:** Inadequate consumption of vital nutrients such as vitamins (e.g., vitamin D, vitamin B12), minerals (e.g., iron, zinc), and protein may damage hair health and contribute to hair loss and thinning during perimenopause. Nutritional deficits may alter the hair development cycle and contribute to thin, brittle hair.

4. **Hormonal Variations:** Hormonal changes, notably variations in oestrogen, progesterone, and testosterone levels, may interrupt the hair development cycle and lead to hair loss and thinning during perimenopause.

5. **Thyroid Disorders:** Thyroid abnormalities, such as hypothyroidism or hyperthyroidism,

may alter the hormonal balance and lead to hair changes during perimenopause. Hypothyroidism, marked by an underactive thyroid gland, may contribute to hair loss, dryness, and thinning.

6. **Drugs and Treatments:** Certain drugs, including hormonal contraceptives, antidepressants, and blood pressure medications, may have adverse effects that include hair loss or thinning. Additionally, therapies such as chemotherapy or radiation therapy for cancer may cause considerable hair loss.

Solutions for Healthy Hair During Perimenopause

1. **Nutritional Support:** Maintain a balanced diet rich in vital nutrients to improve hair health during perimenopause. Incorporate meals abundant in vitamins (e.g., leafy greens, citrus fruits), minerals (e.g., lean meats, legumes), and protein (e.g., fish, eggs) to offer your hair the nutrition it needs to grow.

2. **Supplements:** Consider taking supplements to treat nutritional deficiencies and maintain hair health during perimenopause. Supplements such as biotin, vitamin D, iron, zinc, and omega-3 fatty acids have been demonstrated to boost hair development and prevent hair loss.

3. **Stress Management:** Practise stress-reducing strategies such as meditation, yoga, deep breathing, or mindfulness to limit the influence of stress on hair health during perimenopause. Prioritise self-care activities that promote relaxation and emotional well-being.

4. **Hormone Replacement Therapy (HRT):** Discuss HRT with your healthcare physician as a viable option for addressing hormonal imbalances and accompanying hair changes during perimenopause. HRT may help restore diminishing oestrogen levels and increase hair thickness and growth.

5. **Scalp Care:** Maintain a healthy scalp environment by using mild, sulphate-free

shampoos and avoiding harsh chemicals or excessive heat styling. Incorporate scalp massage methods to boost blood circulation and encourage hair development.

6. **Professional Treatments:** Explore professional hair treatments such as low-level laser therapy (LLLT), platelet-rich plasma (PRP) therapy, or scalp microneedling to stimulate hair follicles and encourage hair growth. Consult with a dermatologist or hair expert to identify the most suitable treatment choices for your unique requirements.

7. **Hair Care Methods:** Adopt hair care methods that minimise damage and breakage, such as using wide-tooth combs, avoiding tight hairstyles, minimising heat styling, and protecting hair from sun exposure and environmental harm.

8. **Consultation with Healthcare Practitioner:** If you notice considerable hair loss or thinning during perimenopause, visit with your healthcare practitioner or a dermatologist to rule out underlying medical

concerns and discuss suitable treatment options. They may make tailored advice based on your specific health history and concerns.

Cosmetic Treatments and Procedures for Hair Loss and Thinning

Hair loss and thinning may severely damage self-esteem and confidence, driving many women to seek cosmetic treatments and surgeries to address these issues. While lifestyle adjustments, hair care practices, and medication interventions may help control hair loss and enhance hair health during perimenopause, cosmetic procedures provide additional alternatives for boosting hair density, thickness, and overall look. Some cosmetic treatments and procedures available for managing hair loss and thinning during perimenopause are:

1. **Scalp Micropigmentation (SMP):** Scalp micropigmentation is a non-invasive cosmetic technique that includes the application of specific pigments to the scalp to produce the appearance of higher hair density. This procedure helps disguise

regions of thinning hair or baldness by duplicating the look of natural hair follicles, giving in a fuller and more uniform scalp appearance.

2. **Hair Transplantation:** Hair transplantation is a surgical treatment that involves removing hair follicles from donor regions (usually the back or sides of the head) and transplanting them into bald or thinning areas of the scalp. This process may efficiently restore hair density and coverage in specified regions, resulting in natural-looking and permanent results.

3. **Platelet-Rich Plasma (PRP) Therapy:** Platelet-rich plasma (PRP) therapy is a non-surgical cosmetic treatment that harnesses the healing qualities of platelets present in the patient's blood to encourage hair growth. During the operation, blood is collected from the patient, processed to separate the platelet-rich plasma, and then injected into the scalp to encourage hair follicle regeneration and development.

4. **Low-Level Laser Therapy (LLLT):** Low-level laser therapy (LLLT), also known as red light therapy or cold laser therapy, is a non-invasive treatment that employs low-level laser devices or caps to stimulate hair follicles and encourage hair growth. LLLT devices emit certain wavelengths of light that are absorbed by the scalp, resulting in enhanced cellular activity and better hair follicle function.

5. **Hair Thickening and Volumizing Products:** Various cosmetic products are available to temporarily increase the appearance of hair thickness and volume. These include volumizing shampoos and conditioners, hair fibres, styling mousses, and volumizing sprays, which may help give the appearance of thicker, fuller hair while providing a temporary covering for areas of thinning.

6. **Topical Hair Growth Therapies:** Topical therapies containing minoxidil, a medicine authorised by the FDA for the treatment of hair loss, may be used directly on the scalp to

promote hair growth and enhance hair density. Minoxidil works by boosting blood flow to the hair follicles and lengthening the growth phase of the hair cycle, resulting in thicker and fuller hair over time.

7. **Hair Extensions and Wigs:** Hair extensions and wigs are non-surgical methods for temporarily improving hair length, volume, and density. Hair extensions are connected to existing hair to improve length and volume, while wigs provide a complete coverage option for ladies facing substantial hair loss or thinning. These solutions give fast results and may be adjusted to fit natural hair colour and texture.

8. **Consultation with a Hair Expert:** Before having any cosmetic treatment or procedure for hair loss or thinning, it's vital to contact a trained hair expert or dermatologist. They may examine your particular requirements and concerns, propose suitable treatment alternatives, and give personalised advise based on your exact hair type, condition, and objectives.

If you are experiencing perimenopause and are beginning to question if your hair is thinning or you are paranoid, don't leave this up to chance, since many women observe the commencement of hair loss around this time. The sooner you address this condition, the more probable it is to be treated.

Chapter 9: Mental Health and Emotional Well-being

As women travel through perimenopause, they manage several physical, hormonal, and psychological changes that may dramatically influence their mental health and emotional well-being. From shifting hormones to managing symptoms such as hot flashes, mood swings, and sleep difficulties, perimenopause brings unique challenges that may take a toll on one's mental health. Understanding these hormone shifts is vital for appreciating their influence on mental health throughout this time.

Impact of Hormonal Changes on Mental Health

Perimenopause is defined by considerable hormonal variations, notably in oestrogen and progesterone levels, which may have dramatic implications on mental health and emotional well-being. These hormonal changes may alter neurotransmitter activity, brain function, and emotional control, leading to a spectrum of psychiatric symptoms and mood problems. Understanding the influence of hormonal changes on mental health is vital for identifying and managing the emotional issues that women may encounter during perimenopause. Let's investigate the numerous ways in which hormone changes might impair mental health during this transitional phase:

1. **Mood Swings and Emotional Lability:** Fluctuating hormone levels, notably oestrogen, and progesterone, may contribute to mood swings and emotional lability during perimenopause. Women may notice rapid fluctuations in mood, ranging from irritation and anxiety to melancholy and tearfulness. These mood variations may be unexpected

and may vary in severity, making it tough to control emotions appropriately.

2. **Increased Chance of Depression:** Hormonal changes during perimenopause might raise the chance of developing depression or intensify current depressed symptoms. Oestrogen plays a vital role in regulating mood, and changes in oestrogen levels during perimenopause may affect serotonin and dopamine neurotransmission, which are important in mood control. Women may suffer emotions of melancholy, despair, worthlessness, and lack of interest or pleasure in things they formerly loved.

3. **Anxiety and Panic Attacks:** Hormonal imbalances, along with stress and life changes associated with perimenopause, may provoke or intensify symptoms of anxiety and panic attacks. Oestrogen variations may impact the activity of neurotransmitters such as gamma-aminobutyric acid (GABA), which modulates anxiety and stress reactions. Women may suffer heightened sensations of concern, dread, restlessness, and physical

symptoms such as palpitations, shortness of breath, and shaking.

4. **Cognitive Changes and Brain Fog:** Hormonal changes during perimenopause may also impair cognitive function and lead to symptoms usually referred to as "brain fog" or cognitive fog. Oestrogen performs a neuroprotective effect in the brain, supporting cognitive functions such as memory, attention, and executive function. Declining oestrogen levels may lead to issues with attention, memory lapses, forgetfulness, and mental sluggishness.

5. **Sleep Disturbances and Insomnia:** Hormonal variations, notably changes in progesterone levels, may disrupt sleep patterns and lead to sleep disturbances and insomnia during perimenopause. Progesterone has calming effects and promotes relaxation, but lowering levels may lead to difficulty falling asleep, staying asleep, or having restorative sleep. Sleep interruptions may increase emotional

disorders, cognitive challenges, and general well-being.

6. **Impact on Stress Response and Coping Mechanisms:** Hormonal changes during perimenopause might impact the body's stress response system and coping mechanisms, affecting how women perceive and react to stresses. Oestrogen and progesterone perform functions in influencing the hypothalamic-pituitary-adrenal (HPA) axis, which modulates the stress response. Dysregulation of the HPA axis may result in heightened stress sensitivity, maladaptive coping techniques, and greater susceptibility to stress-related mental health disorders.

7. **Relationship with Menopausal issues:** Mental health issues during perimenopause are typically intermingled with physical menopausal symptoms such as hot flashes, night sweats, and vaginal dryness. The feeling of psychological anguish may increase physical symptoms, whereas physical pain can lead to emotional distress

and adversely influence mental health outcomes.

Coping Strategies for Supporting Mental Well-being

1. **Hormone Balancing Approaches:** Consult with a naturopathic practitioner skilled in women's health to investigate natural ways of hormone balancing. Herbal medicines, dietary assistance, and lifestyle adjustments targeted to your unique requirements may help reduce symptoms and enhance mental well-being.

2. **Stress Management and Relaxation Techniques:** Stress might increase perimenopausal symptoms. Incorporate stress reduction strategies like meditation, deep breathing exercises, and mindfulness practices into your daily routine to build emotional resilience.

3. **Prioritise Self-Care:** Make self-care a non-negotiable priority. Engage in things that offer you pleasure, lower stress levels, and

encourage relaxation. Nourish your body with healthy food, prioritise excellent sleep, and practice self-compassion.

4. **Seek Support:** Don't hesitate to seek out healthcare specialists or therapists specialised in menopause-related mental health. They can give information, coping skills, and support targeted to your requirements.

5. **Connect with Others:** Building a support network of women living through perimenopause may create a feeling of community and understanding. Share experiences, worries, and thoughts in online forums, support groups, or local menopause-focused communities.

Perimenopause is a journey packed with unique difficulties and changes, not just on a medical level but also in terms of mental well-being. Understanding the dance of hormones during this era helps you to negotiate the ups and downs with strength and grace. By applying measures for maintaining mental health, obtaining expert help, and practising self-care, you may face this transitional time with confidence and emerge stronger on the other side.

Chapter 10: Sleep and Fatigue Management for Perimenopausal Women

Sleep problems and exhaustion are typical complaints among women undergoing perimenopause, reducing general well-being and quality of life. The hormonal swings and physiological changes that occur during this transitional period might disturb sleep habits, resulting in problems falling asleep, staying asleep, or reaching restorative sleep. Additionally, hormone imbalances and lifestyle variables may lead to sensations of sleepiness and exhaustion, further complicating sleep-related disorders.

In this chapter, we will investigate the complicated relationship between perimenopause, sleep, and tiredness, offering insights into the underlying reasons for sleep disruptions and weariness during this time of life.

Impact of Hormonal Changes on Sleep Patterns

Oestrogen, progesterone, and other hormones play critical roles in regulating the sleep-wake cycle, encouraging restful sleep, and maintaining general sleep health. However, when women approach menopause, fluctuations in hormone levels may disrupt these regulating processes, leading to sleep disorders and insomnia. The following are some influences of hormonal changes on sleep patterns during perimenopause:

1. **Oestrogen Decline:** Oestrogen, a crucial reproductive hormone, regulates sleep architecture and quality by altering neurotransmitters and receptors involved in sleep regulation. As oestrogen levels diminish during perimenopause, women may suffer disturbances in sleep patterns, including trouble falling asleep, numerous awakenings throughout the night, and overall lower sleep quality.

2. **Progesterone Fluctuations:** Progesterone, another hormone involved in menstrual cycle control, also plays a function in sleep modulation and relaxation. Fluctuations in progesterone levels during perimenopause might lead to sleep disorders, such as insomnia, restless legs syndrome, and fragmented sleep.

3. **Impact on Circadian Rhythm:** Hormonal changes during perimenopause might disturb the body's internal clock, known as the circadian rhythm, which governs the sleep-wake cycle. Alterations in circadian rhythm may lead to changes in sleep time, inconsistent sleep patterns, and difficulties maintaining normal sleep-wake cycles, further worsening sleep disorders.

4. **Vasomotor Symptoms:** Vasomotor symptoms, such as hot flashes and night sweats, are frequent during perimenopause and may greatly disturb sleep continuity and quality. Fluctuations in hormone levels, especially oestrogen, are likely to contribute

to the prevalence and severity of vasomotor symptoms, resulting in sleep fragmentation and nocturnal awakenings.

5. **Mood and Stress:** Hormonal changes during perimenopause may impair mood regulation and stress responses, leading to heightened emotional reactivity and psychological suffering. Mood disorders, such as anxiety and depression, are related to sleep abnormalities, including trouble falling asleep, early morning awakenings, and non-restorative sleep.

6. **Sleep-Disordered Breathing:** Changes in hormone levels during perimenopause may potentially alter respiratory function and raise the risk of sleep-disordered breathing disorders, including obstructive sleep apnea (OSA). OSA is marked by recurring bouts of partial or total airway blockage during sleep, resulting in altered sleep patterns and daytime weariness.

7. **Hormone Replacement Therapy (HRT):** HRT, which includes the injection of

oestrogen, progesterone, or a combination of both hormones, may alter sleep patterns and quality in women experiencing perimenopause. HRT may reduce vasomotor symptoms and enhance sleep continuity, however, its effects on sleep may vary based on individual characteristics and treatment regimes.

8. **Impact on Sleep Architecture:** Hormonal changes during perimenopause might modify sleep architecture, influencing the distribution and length of distinct sleep phases, including slow-wave sleep (deep sleep) and rapid eye movement (REM) sleep. Disruptions in sleep architecture may lead to non-restorative sleep and daytime drowsiness.

Proven Strategies for Improving Sleep Quality

Despite how crucial sleep is to physical and mental well-being, you may find it tough to obtain enough quality sleep each night. The consequences of inadequate sleep may be seen in many aspects of your life.

Managing sleep disruptions and enhancing sleep quality during perimenopause is vital for supporting general health and well-being. Through the application of effective tactics and lifestyle adjustments, women may improve their sleep hygiene and boost the quality of their restorative sleep. Here are some ways to enhance sleep quality during perimenopause:

1. **Establish a Consistent Sleep Schedule:** Maintain a consistent sleep-wake routine by going to bed and getting up at the same time every day, especially on weekends. Consistency helps regulate your body's internal clock and promotes improved sleep quality.

2. **Create a Relaxing Nighttime Ritual:** Develop a peaceful nighttime ritual to communicate to your body that it's time to wind down and prepare for sleep. Activities like reading, listening to calming music, having a warm bath, or practising relaxation methods may assist in inducing relaxation and lower stress levels before sleep.

3. **Create a Comfortable Sleep Environment:** Make your bedroom favourable to sleep by adjusting environmental aspects such as temperature, lighting, and noise levels. Keep your bedroom cold, dark, and quiet to produce an optimal sleep environment that promotes relaxation and regenerative sleep.

4. **Invest in a Supportive Mattress and Pillows:** Choose a comfortable mattress and supportive pillows that give enough support for your body and encourage good spinal alignment. A quality sleep surface may increase sleep comfort and lessen the chance of discomfort or pain that may disturb sleep.

5. **Limit Stimulants and Electronics Before Bed:** Avoid ingesting stimulants such as coffee and nicotine in the hours preceding bedtime, since they may interfere with sleep onset and quality. Additionally, minimise exposure to electronic devices such as cellphones, tablets, and laptops, since the blue light generated from displays may disrupt melatonin synthesis and impair sleep.

6. **Practice Stress Reduction Tactics:** Incorporate stress reduction tactics into your everyday routine to reduce tension and promote relaxation. Techniques such as deep breathing exercises, progressive muscle relaxation, mindfulness meditation, or yoga may help quiet the mind and body before bedtime, promoting greater sleep quality.

7. **Limit Daytime Naps:** Limit daytime napping to prevent disturbing your normal sleep-wake cycle and promote improved nightly sleep quality. If you feel the desire to sleep throughout the day, keep it brief (20-30 minutes) and avoid resting too close to bedtime.

8. **Regular Exercise:** Engage in regular physical activity, such as aerobic exercise, yoga, or walking, to support better sleep quality and general health. Regular exercise may help decrease stress, regulate hormones, and enhance sleep efficiency.

9. **Consider Cognitive Behavioral Therapy for Insomnia (CBT-I):** If you encounter chronic insomnia or persistent sleep difficulties, consider obtaining help from a sleep expert or therapist specialised in cognitive-behavioural therapy for insomnia (CBT-I). CBT-I is a systematic, evidence-based method that tackles underlying sleep-related behaviours, beliefs, and routines to enhance sleep quality and quantity.

10. **Pay Attention to What You Eat and Drink:** Don't go to bed hungry or full. In particular, avoid heavy or substantial meals within a couple of hours before sleep. Discomfort could keep you awake. Nicotine, coffee, and alcohol demand prudence, too. The energising effects of nicotine and caffeine take hours to wear off and might interfere with sleep. And although alcohol could help you feel drowsy at first, it might disturb sleep later in the night.

11. **Manage Anxieties:** Try to address your worries or concerns before sleep. Jot down

what's on your mind and then lay it away for tomorrow.

Stress management could assist. Start with the fundamentals, such as becoming organised, defining priorities, and delegating chores. Meditation also helps alleviate anxiety.

12. **Minimise Noise:** Keeping noise to a minimum is a crucial aspect of constructing a sleep-friendly environment. If you cannot remove local sources of noise, try drowning them out with a fan or white noise generator. Earplugs or headphones are another alternative to block noises from annoying you while you want to sleep.

13. **Block Out Light:** Excess light exposure might throw off your sleep and circadian cycle. Blackout curtains over your windows or a sleep mask over your eyes may filter light and prevent it from interfering with your relaxation. Avoiding bright light may help you transition to nighttime and contribute to your body's synthesis of melatonin, a hormone that promotes sleep.

14. **Monitor and Manage Menopausal Symptoms:** Make efforts to manage menopausal symptoms such as hot flashes, night sweats, and mood problems, since these may dramatically impair sleep quality. Talk to your healthcare practitioner about treatment choices, lifestyle adjustments, and coping methods to ease symptoms and enhance sleep.

Relaxation Techniques and Sleep Aids for Improved Sleeping

Relaxation methods and sleep aids may play a crucial role in encouraging restful sleep and treating sleep problems during perimenopause. Here are several relaxing strategies and sleep aids to assist you attain improved sleep quality during perimenopause:

1. **Mindfulness Meditation:** Mindfulness meditation entails concentrating your attention on the present moment without judgement, enabling you to build awareness and acceptance of your thoughts, emotions,

and physiological sensations. Practising mindfulness meditation before bedtime may help calm the mind, decrease racing thoughts, and induce relaxation conducive to sleep.

Progressive Muscle Relaxation (PMR) Progressive muscle relaxation is a method that includes gradually tensing and relaxing various muscle groups in the body to reduce tension and generate a state of profound relaxation. By systematically relaxing each muscle group, beginning from your toes and working your way up to your head, you may induce physical and mental relaxation, making it easier to fall asleep.

2. **Deep Breathing Exercises:** Deep breathing exercises, such as diaphragmatic breathing or 4-7-8 breathing, use slow, deep inhalations and exhalations to activate the body's relaxation response and lower stress levels. By concentrating on your breath and managing your breathing patterns, you may quiet your nervous system, reduce cortisol levels, and induce feelings of relaxation conducive to sleep.

3. **Guided Imagery and Visualization:** Guided imagery and visualisation methods entail mentally visualising pleasant and relaxing surroundings, such as a placid beach or tranquil forest, to elicit emotions of relaxation and calmness. By immersing yourself in vivid and sensory-rich images, you may divert your mind from problems and pressures, encouraging a feeling of tranquillity and preparation for sleep.

4. **Yoga and Stretching:** Practising simple yoga postures and stretching activities before sleep may help relieve tension from the body, decrease muscular stiffness, and promote relaxation. Incorporate moderate yoga sequences, such as restorative yoga or nighttime yoga, to gently stretch and relax your muscles, preparing your body for comfortable sleep.

5. **Aromatherapy:** Aromatherapy includes utilising essential oils with relaxing and soothing characteristics, such as lavender, chamomile, or bergamot, to encourage

relaxation and enhance sleep quality. Diffuse essential oils in your bedroom, add a few drops to a warm bath, or apply them topically to pulse points to experience their relaxing benefits before sleep.

6. **White Noise and Relaxing Sounds:** White noise generators, natural sounds, or peaceful music may produce a pleasant auditory environment that conceals external disturbances and promotes relaxation favourable to sleep. Experiment with various noises and frequencies to determine what works best for you and increases your sleep quality.

7. **Sleep Aids and Supplements:** Consider utilising sleep aids and supplements, such as melatonin, valerian root, or magnesium, to help relax and increase sleep quality. These natural therapies may help manage sleep-wake cycles, increase relaxation, and shorten the time it takes to fall asleep.

Fatigue Management and Energy Levels: Diet and Nutrition

Fatigue is a typical symptom during perimenopause, generally ascribed to hormone imbalances, sleep difficulties, and lifestyle factors. While treating underlying causes of exhaustion is vital, adopting a balanced diet and integrating particular nutrients may help improve energy levels and counteract symptoms of weariness and lethargy. Here's a look at how food and nutrition may play a significant part in reducing tiredness and increasing sustained energy levels during perimenopause:

1. **Balanced Macronutrient Intake:** Consume a balanced diet that contains enough quantities of carbs, proteins, and healthy fats to give sustained energy throughout the day. Carbohydrates are the body's major source of energy and should be acquired from whole grains, fruits, vegetables, and legumes. Pair carbs with lean proteins and healthy fats to regulate blood sugar levels and avoid energy dips.

2. **Complex Carbohydrates:** Choose complex carbohydrates with a low glycemic index, such as whole grains (oats, quinoa, brown rice), legumes (beans, lentils), and starchy vegetables (sweet potatoes, squash), which give a consistent release of energy and help maintain stable blood sugar levels. Avoid simple carbs and processed sugars, which may contribute to energy spikes and crashes.

3. **Protein-Rich Foods:** Include lean sources of protein in your diet, such as chicken, fish, tofu, beans, lentils, eggs, and dairy products, to assist muscle repair and energy generation. Protein helps regulate blood sugar levels, induce fullness, and reduce energy dips between meals.

4. **Healthy Fats:** Incorporate sources of healthy fats, such as avocados, nuts, seeds, olive oil, and fatty fish (salmon, mackerel, sardines), into your diet to give long-lasting energy and boost brain function. Healthy fats are needed for hormone synthesis, cell membrane function, and energy metabolism.

5. **Hydration:** Stay hydrated throughout the day by consuming a suitable quantity of water, herbal teas, and electrolyte-rich drinks to avoid dehydration, which may lead to sensations of exhaustion and lethargy. Aim to drink at least eight glasses of water every day, and vary your fluid intake depending on activity level and ambient circumstances.

6. **Nutrient-Dense Foods:** Focus on nutrient-dense foods that contain critical vitamins, minerals, and antioxidants to enhance overall health and energy levels. Incorporate a range of colourful fruits and vegetables, leafy greens, nuts, seeds, and whole grains into your meals to ensure you're fulfilling your nutritional requirements and boosting optimum energy production.

7. **Balanced Meals and Snacks:** Plan balanced meals and snacks that contain a variety of carbs, proteins, and healthy fats to offer sustained energy throughout the day. Aim for smaller, frequent meals and snacks to reduce energy dips and stabilise blood sugar levels.

8. **Limit Caffeine and Sugar:** Limit the use of caffeine and sugary drinks, since they may produce brief energy increases followed by crashes and exhaustion. Opt for caffeine-free herbal teas, sparkling water, or green tea for hydration, and pick naturally sweetened snacks, such as fresh fruit or yoghourt, to fulfil cravings without increasing blood sugar levels.

9. **Time of Meals:** Pay attention to the time of your meals and snacks to minimise energy slumps and encourage maintained energy levels. Aim for frequent meals and snacks spaced evenly throughout the day to maintain stable blood sugar levels and minimise overeating or undereating, which may impair energy levels.

10. **Nutritional Supplements:** Consider introducing nutritional supplements, such as vitamin B complex, iron, magnesium, and coenzyme Q10, into your daily routine to enhance energy generation, minimise tiredness, and improve overall well-being. Consult with a healthcare physician or trained

dietitian to decide whether supplementation is appropriate depending on your unique requirements and health state.

Stress Management and Restorative Practices

Perimenopause may be a hard period defined by hormonal shifts, physical symptoms, and emotional changes, all of which can lead to heightened stress levels. Effective stress management is key for sustaining general well-being and navigating through this time with resilience and vigour. Adding stress management strategies and restorative practices into your daily routine may help decrease tension, improve relaxation, and boost your capacity to deal with the problems of perimenopause. Here's a guide on stress management and restorative activities especially for women going through perimenopause:

1. **Yoga and Tai Chi:** Yoga and tai chi are mind-body practices that integrate gentle movements, breathwork, and mindfulness to improve relaxation, flexibility, and stress reduction. Engage in frequent yoga or tai chi

sessions to lower stress levels, boost mood, and promote general well-being during perimenopause.

2. **Nature Therapy (Forest Bathing):** Spend time in nature and immerse yourself in natural settings to enjoy the therapeutic advantages of forest bathing. Nature therapy, often known as forest bathing, may decrease stress hormones, lower blood pressure, and enhance mood, giving a natural antidote to the strains of everyday life.

3. **Creative Expression:** Engage in creative hobbies such as painting, sketching, writing, or crafts to express oneself artistically and reduce stress. Creative expression may serve as a type of self-care, enabling you to channel your emotions, ideas, and experiences into meaningful and therapeutic outlets.

4. **Journaling and Reflection:** Keep a journal to examine your ideas, emotions, and experiences throughout perimenopause, allowing for self-reflection and emotional processing. Writing may serve as a

therapeutic avenue for expressing feelings, acquiring insights, and growing self-awareness.

5. **Social help and Connection:** Seek help from friends, family members, or support groups who understand and sympathise with your experiences throughout perimenopause. Social support and connection may give emotional affirmation, practical aid, and a feeling of belonging, buffering against the negative consequences of stress.

6. **Healthy Lifestyle Habits:** Prioritise healthy lifestyle habits such as frequent exercise, balanced eating, appropriate sleep, and water to improve general well-being and resistance to stress. Engage in things that offer you pleasure and contentment, establishing a feeling of purpose and meaning in life.

7. **Professional Help:** If stress becomes overwhelming or interferes with your everyday functioning, get professional help from a therapist, counsellor, or healthcare practitioner. Therapy may give coping

methods, emotional support, and assistance for managing stress and navigating through perimenopause with better comfort.

In addition, stress has been well proven to aggravate physical and mental perimenopause symptoms. In particular vasomotor symptoms such as hot flashes and night sweats occur higher for women who suffer discomfort from stressful life/events. Meditation and mindfulness-based stress reduction (MBSR) are both beneficial ways of controlling stress during perimenopause. Meditation is effective in lowering anxiety and mood problems.

Women practising mindfulness-based stress reduction (MBSR) in a randomised controlled experiment had less depressive symptoms, less perceived stress, less anxiety, higher resilience, and improved sleep

Chapter 11: Conclusion: Embracing the Journey of Perimenopause

As we reach the culmination of this transformative journey through perimenopause, it's essential to reflect on the myriad experiences, challenges, and triumphs that have shaped our path. From the subtle shifts in our bodies to the profound fluctuations in our emotions, perimenopause has been a rollercoaster ride of change, growth, and self-discovery. As we bid farewell to this chapter of our lives, let us pause to celebrate the resilience, strength, and wisdom that have carried us through the peaks and valleys of this transitional phase.

Throughout this book, we've embarked on a comprehensive exploration of perimenopause, delving into its multifaceted dimensions and uncovering the intricate interplay of hormones, symptoms, and lifestyle factors that define this stage of life. From understanding the physiological mechanisms driving hormonal changes to navigating the myriad symptoms that accompany perimenopause, we've equipped ourselves with knowledge, insight, and practical strategies to empower us on our journey.

We've delved into the intricacies of hormonal fluctuations, exploring their impact on physical health, mental well-being, and emotional balance. We've navigated the maze of menopausal symptoms, from hot flashes and night sweats to mood swings and sleep disturbances, with resilience and grace. We've embraced self-care practices, from mindful meditation and yoga to nutrition and sleep hygiene, to nourish our bodies, minds, and spirits.

We've emphasised the importance of seeking support, whether from healthcare providers, therapists, or trusted friends and family members, to navigate the challenges of perimenopause with courage and resilience. We've fostered a community of solidarity and empowerment, offering compassion, understanding, and encouragement to one another as we journey through this transitional phase together.

As we bid farewell to perimenopause and embrace the next chapter of our lives, let us carry forward the lessons learned, the insights gained, and the connections forged along the way. Let us continue to nurture our bodies, minds, and spirits with compassion, kindness, and self-love. And let us embrace the journey ahead with open hearts, curious minds, and unwavering resilience.

For in the tapestry of our lives, perimenopause is but one thread, woven seamlessly into the fabric of our womanhood. And as we emerge on the other side, we emerge stronger, wiser, and more radiant than ever before. So let us embrace the beauty of this transformative journey, for it is in the journey itself that we find our truest selves and our deepest purpose.

Congratulations and thank you for reading through!

Feedback

Dear Valued Readers,

As I reflect on the journey we've embarked on together through the pages of this book, I'm filled with gratitude for the opportunity to share insights, knowledge, and experiences on the topic of perimenopause. Your support and engagement have been the driving force behind this endeavour, and I am truly humbled by the trust you've placed in me as an author.

As I strive to continually improve and evolve in my craft, I recognize the invaluable role that feedback and reviews play in shaping future publications. Your honest insights, reflections, and critiques provide invaluable guidance and inspiration, guiding me towards creating content that resonates deeply with you, my cherished readers.

I invite you to share your thoughts, opinions, and feedback on this book through a review on online platforms. Your input is invaluable in helping me understand what resonated with you, what areas could be further explored, and how I can better serve you in future publications.

Additionally, I would like to extend an invitation for you to connect with me on my Author Central account. By following me on Author Central, you'll receive prompt notifications whenever I release new publications, allowing you to stay informed about upcoming releases, exclusive content, and special offers.

Your feedback fuels my passion for writing and empowers me to continue striving for excellence in delivering content that informs, inspires, and uplifts.

Thank you for your unwavering support, your candid feedback, and your commitment to the pursuit of knowledge and understanding. I look forward to hearing from you, connecting with you on Author Central, and embarking on future journeys together.

With heartfelt gratitude,

Kristin Hampton

Recommendation

If you are looking for a way to overcome dull, lacklustre skin that leaves you feeling less than confident, or if you're seeking solutions to maintain a healthy lifestyle amidst the demands of daily life, then this book is your answer.

Packed with practical tips and expert advice, it offers a comprehensive guide to achieving radiant skin, vibrant health, and holistic wellness. Say goodbye to skincare woes and health concerns, and hello to a more confident, balanced you.
Don't let another day go by without taking control of your well-being - get a copy now through the link below or search for the title now.

https://www.amazon.com/dp/B0CVQCB3WQ

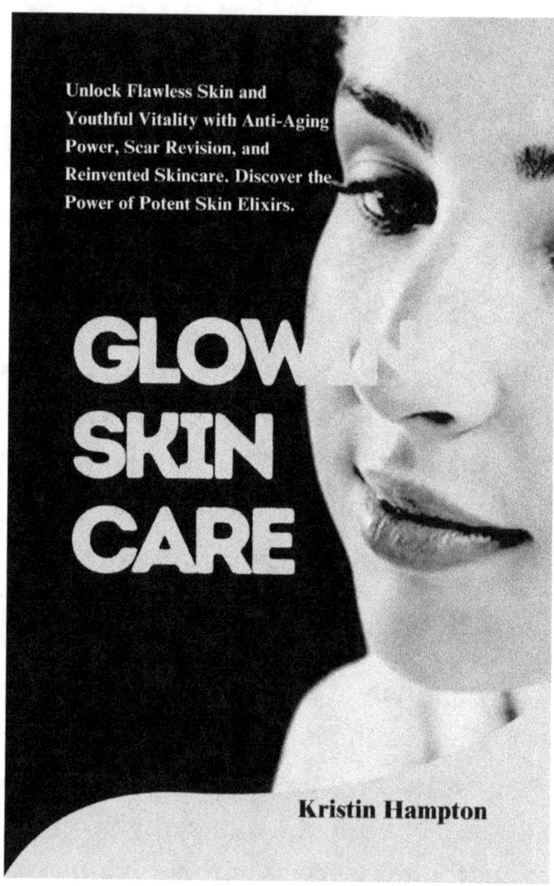